Putting Our House
in Order

Contents

Preface

THIS BOOK GOT ITS START from a luncheon conversation. We talked about the sense of unease that characterizes much of the writing about the future of the American economy. The unease is produced by a feeling that the costs of entitlement programs—Social Security, Medicare, and Medicaid—are out of control and will overwhelm the budget. That will bring a catastrophe for beneficiaries whose needs will not be served and for the fiscal stability of the United States. Something, we agreed, needs fixing so that people can be confident that reasonable benefits will be there for them and that the economy will remain healthy.

Anyone can see that the entitlement problems need to be solved. Is it possible? As we tackled this subject, we felt more and more convinced that the problems are soluble, at least in concept. Whether or not the political process can work out sensible changes is certainly an open question, but we are confident that progress can be made by reaffirming the wide consensus that present programs are not sustainable and by showing that there are workable alternatives.

We received a great deal of help in developing our ideas. We talked to colleagues and exploited their patience and goodwill, as well as their knowledge. Paul Berg, Michael Boskin, John Cogan, Victor Fuchs, Greg Rosston, and John Taylor read an early draft of the book and made comments that were very helpful. Vidar Jorgensen suggested materials in the health care area for us to consider. Susan Southworth has managed the manuscript through umpteen drafts with skill and care and has given us the benefit of her editing talent. Drake McFeely, with his editorial and organizational suggestions and his perspective derived from years of success in the publishing world, has been a masterful commentator.

We are deeply grateful for all this help. At the same time, if any reader has an argument, argue with us, not them.

Introduction

THE UNITED STATES faces the daunting imperative of identifying solutions to manage the staggering projected costs of its Social Security, Medicaid, and Medicare systems, our so-called entitlement programs. The magnitude of these costs cannot be met by any reasonable projection of future federal government revenues. The U.S. body politic must somehow find a way to ensure that systems are in place to provide reasonable income for the elderly and universal access to health care that are consistent with fiscal sanity. The purpose of this book is to help find a way to make progress on this most important problem.

When Ben Bernanke, the chairman of the Federal Reserve Board, was asked by the Senate Budget Committee when the problems of Social Security, Medicare, and Medicaid would need to be addressed, he replied, "I think the right time to start is about ten years ago."[1]

Our approach differs from the theme of impending catastrophe in much of the current writing about the

U.S. economy. Two recent publications tell the story in their titles: *Running on Empty* by Peter G. Peterson, and "Is the United States Bankrupt?" by Laurence J. Kotlikoff.[2] Both are informed, responsible wake-up calls, and they have plenty of company. Careful projections of future costs made by the Congressional Budget Office (CBO), for example, show that entitlement costs alone could reach 28.5 percent of gross domestic product by 2050, clearly an unmanageable level, especially considering that federal revenues have never exceeded 21 percent of GDP in the history of the Republic.[3] And these projections reveal only part of the problems before us. Commitments by state and city governments and by private employers contribute substantially to the looming threat described in chapter 2, "The Iceberg Ahead."

Clearly, something needs to be done, but this difficult subject merits a positive approach. America's solid record of economic achievement holds the promise of continued success in a future filled with opportunity. American success exists on many fronts. The U.S. economy sets the world standard, and its growth is an essential ingredient in the expanding global economy. The creativity and dynamism of the American economy now yield strong gains in productivity (output per man-hour) that surpass the rate of improvement in many prior decades. The U.S. economy produces one of the highest per capita incomes in the world, and no other major developed country has been able to keep pace, let alone catch up. So it's clear: We have success on our hands.

And the economy is by no means the only area of success. Not only do Americans live longer than ever before, but many are healthier and capable of being productive far longer than at any time in the past. These trends are likely to continue as a result of many breathtaking advances in science and technology. Such momentous developments are opportunities to nourish.

The contradiction between this clear evidence of success and the current atmosphere of unease in the United States calls for a change in mind-set. The projected gargantuan shortfalls in the U.S. budget stem largely from the interaction of constantly expanding costs of health care and longer life spans with relatively inflexible entitlement programs. Increasing longevity and better health are developments to celebrate. The challenge is to adapt income support and health care programs to these changing demographics and health care options.

The difficult problems of financing Social Security and health care commitments must be approached from a realistic perspective based on demography, medical developments, and fundamental economics. In demographic terms, we are retiring earlier and living longer. The result is a growing proportion of people outside the labor force compared with those who are working. Medical treatment options too have expanded. As a consequence, the federal government has increasingly become a mechanism for transferring ever-mounting sums of money from younger workers to older retired Americans.

Solutions to the entitlement problems will be made easier or more difficult according to the size and rate of growth of GDP, so the first step toward seizing opportunities is the promotion of a large, growing economy. That means examining those characteristics that strengthen the U.S. economy and addressing those that need to be stronger. Any reforms of entitlement programs should be consistent with these objectives. In addition, this book will look at ways in which the structure of retirement and health systems can be changed to improve participation in the labor force and to increase the rate of private saving. Labor and capital, after all, are the primary inputs that create GDP.

The history of Social Security and health care programs in the United States shows that their structural roots come from an altogether different era, that of the Great Depression and World War II and its aftermath. These programs must be adjusted to better accommodate increased longevity as well as improved and promising medical treatments, which are often costly.

The Social Security system was part of President Franklin D. Roosevelt's New Deal. First enacted in 1935 and changed many times since then, this program provides a base of income support for the elderly and is financed by a tax on labor earnings. Since revenues from taxes on current workers pay for the retirement income of those eligible to draw benefits, the program's financing structure is known as pay-as-you-go.

Federal government support for access to the health care system started during World War II, when wages were controlled and heavily taxed. The provision of health insurance, which was neither controlled nor taxed, was an important way for employers to compete for scarce labor, so the use of these plans exploded. The dominance of employment-provided health insurance continues to this day. The initial structure of these plans put the employee in the position of having tax-free access to health care services without any out-of-pocket cost. Not surprisingly under these circumstances, use increased sharply.

In 1965 government involvement in the health care area expanded dramatically. Medicare provided access to benefits for those over sixty-five years of age, and Medicaid provided access, in the form of federal-state programs, for the poor. These programs have become more complex as they have evolved over the years. Nevertheless, their essential structure, like the employer insurance model, initially provided mostly free services to those eligible, or "entitled," to receive them.

Reform of these programs will not come easily. To touch them, many politicians worry, is to touch a third rail. But well-documented projections of the costs of current programs show that inaction is simply not an option. Progress will be promoted by widespread realization of the depth of the problem and of the fact that workable options exist. In fact, the rigidity and stability of the programs are major parts of the problem. Everything about the U.S. economy is dynamic except its major entitlement programs. To serve their fundamental purposes, these programs must be modernized so that they are suitable for the twenty-first century. We shall present several proposals for reforming these important aspects of the economy along with our own recommendations, developed to meet the tests of fairness and fiscal responsibility.

PART ONE

Perspectives

CHAPTER ONE

A Story of Success:
Healthy People in a
Healthy Economy

ED WHITLOCK, a seventy-three-year-old marathoner, broke his own record in September 2004 at the Toronto Waterfront Marathon.[1] He ran the distance of 26 miles 385 yards in 2:54:49, placing twenty-sixth among 1,690 finishers and setting the world record for runners over seventy years of age. Whitlock has company. Among the United States' 400,000 marathon finishers in 2003, approximately 500 were older than seventy compared with about 100 a decade earlier. The National Institutes of Health has interesting ideas about why older people can achieve greater health and fitness gains from exercise than previously thought. In fact, health statistics are consistent with Whitlock's performance: They show that the chances of living a long, healthy life are steadily improving.

Increasing longevity, the most basic measure of health, is a phenomenon in the United States that is apparent at almost any age. Rightly or wrongly, sixty-five is the commonly accepted line between middle age and old age. In 1935, when the Social Security system was established, life expectancy of males and females at age sixty-five was twelve and thirteen years respectively. But life expectancy for men at age sixty-five has increased by 35 percent since then (to sixteen years in 2004), and by 43 percent for women (to nineteen years in 2004).[2] In fact, male life expectancy at age sixty-five has been growing by about one month per year for the past thirty years or so. Every year, new cohorts of Social Security and Medicare participants live one month longer, on average, than the previous year's groups.

A related point is that the fraction of male Medicare enrollees aged sixty-five or older who are chronically disabled declined by 20 percent from 1984 to 1999.[3] In other words, not only has longevity increased, but individuals aged sixty-five and older are healthier than in the past. In effect, they are "younger" than were people of the same age decades earlier.

Increasing life expectancy is a worldwide phenomenon, and many population experts believe that longevity in the United States is likely to increase more rapidly than the Social Security Administration's current predictions. The fact that life expectancy in Japan is approximately four years higher than in the United States indicates that further progress in the average length of life of Americans is perfectly feasible.

Venture capitalists and pharmaceutical companies are betting on this trend by investing billions of dollars in biogenetics. Many in the medical community share their optimism. Scientific research and development have produced an increasing array of medications, medical procedures and instruments, and an understanding of human health, all of which have made dramatic contributions to the length and quality of life. There is every reason to expect that these developments will continue and that many of the investments being made will pay off.

Improvements in health include a sharp decline in deaths and disabilities caused by heart disease over the last two decades or so. Primary credit for this decline goes to new drugs developed to control high blood pressure and high cholesterol. If heart disease continues to decline, and if significant progress is made in the treatment of cancer and Alzheimer's disease, the average length of life will increase, quite likely by an amount larger than that reflected in official government projections.

Health education and economic incentives have contributed to these improvements in health and longevity. As smoking has been linked increasingly to a wide variety of debilitating diseases, antitobacco campaigns have been launched, and cigarette taxes have risen steadily. The result is a sharp fall in the number of men aged sixty-five and over who smoke cigarettes. The number of female smokers over age sixty-five, traditionally much smaller than that of male smokers, has also declined in recent years.[4]

On the other hand, obesity presents an increasing health problem for children and adults, and some population experts believe that life expectancy gains may slow as obesity takes its toll. The percentage of men aged sixty-five to seventy-four who are obese has jumped from 10 percent to 25 percent over the last forty years, and the picture is even more dismal for women.[5] The adverse impact of obesity on health has been somewhat muted by new medications for high blood pressure, excessive cholesterol levels, and diabetes, yet it is still a serious national health problem.

Nevertheless, the overall picture in the United States is one of improving health for individuals in all age-groups. This is borne out by the positive self-assessments gathered from the general population. For example, two-thirds of non-Hispanic whites who are eighty-five years and older describe their own health as good to excellent, and other groups are nearly as optimistic.[6]

Today men and women in the United States live longer and healthier lives than at any time in the past. The clear expectation is that this positive trend will continue. Hand in hand with such success comes the need to manage retirement and health care policies responsibly.

The Strong Economy of the United States

An aging and healthy population will cause the output of the U.S. economy to shift in the direction of the elderly. How can this change be managed? Think of the

U.S. economy as a large pie, and consider the problem of dividing that pie between those who are hard at work producing it, today's labor force, and those who helped create it but no longer contribute to its size and composition, retirees. Division is always difficult. Initially most people seem to focus instinctively on financial systems—entitlement programs—that accomplish this division automatically. But consider a different approach. The most important objective should be to ensure that the size of the pie continues to grow as time goes on. An ever-expanding pie eases the tough choices of allocating shares between today's labor force and those who have retired.

A large and growing pie requires a substantial workforce with a high and rising rate of productivity. So the first step in addressing the issues posed by the prospective costs of income for retirees and health expenditures for everyone, most especially for those who have retired, is to identify the strengths and weaknesses of the U.S. economy and make suggestions for their improvement. The story begins with the stability of the economy.

Over the last 150 years the U.S. economy has become increasingly stable. The economy was in recession nearly 45 percent of the time during the last half of the nineteenth century, 33 percent in the first half of the twentieth century, and 16 percent in the last half of the twentieth century. In the post–World War II period, the occurrence of down quarters has diminished from sixteen in the years between 1946 to 1965 to fifteen from 1966 to 1985 to just five since then. Meanwhile, even as the economy has grown to Herculean size, its real rate of growth has continued to be robust. In the last twenty-five years, the real growth rate averaged 3.1 percent, maintaining the average level of the post–World War II period. The slowing growth rate in our population, hence in labor force expansion, will cause economic growth to moderate somewhat in the years ahead. Nevertheless, this impressive progress gives a sense of what is possible in the future. For example, if the average growth rate of the last twenty years prevails for the next twenty, the present U.S. economy of $13 trillion will grow to nearly $25 trillion.

The last twenty-five-year period has also been one of relatively stable prices, with the inflation rate being substantially below 4 percent on a sustained basis. In post–World War II history, only the period beginning around 1950 is comparable, although its rate of economic growth was lower than that of the last quarter century. Moreover, inflation soared from the late 1960s through most of the 1970s, and by 1980 it was running at about 14 percent, a rate that brought about the sustained effort to control inflation that has been at work for the last twenty-five years. The resulting predictability of price levels has contributed to investment and thus to economic growth. The lesson is clear: A monetary policy that is compatible with a low, stable rate of inflation is essential to a healthy and growing economy.

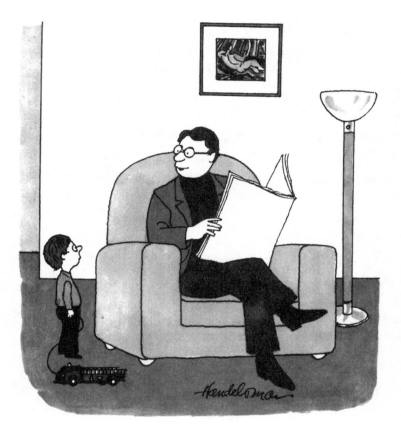

"By the way, Sam, as someday you'll be paying for my entitlements, I'd like to thank you in advance."

Changes in the structure and level of taxation have also been important contributors to a healthy economy. Top marginal tax rates declined dramatically between 1960 and 1986, as shown in chart 1.1. Note that until 2003 the top marginal tax rates on ordinary income and dividends were one and the same. Today it is hard to imagine that as recently as 1961, when President John F. Kennedy took office, the top marginal rate of taxation was 91 percent. Kennedy boldly initiated rate reductions that fully materialized during the Johnson years, bringing the top rate down to 70 percent, although it increased again because of the surtax to finance the Vietnam War in the later years of the Johnson administration. The rate subsequently declined again to 70 percent and stayed at that level throughout the Nixon, Ford, and Carter administrations.

Then came the Reagan years. Early in his presidency Ronald Reagan persuaded Congress to reduce the top tax rate from 70 percent to 50 percent. Then, in 1986, in a dramatic, bipartisan piece of legislation, revenues were increased by stripping loopholes and preferences out of the tax law and then commensurably decreased by reducing the top marginal rate to 28 percent. The result was that the 1986 tax reform was revenue neutral. The top marginal tax rate inched back up again by 3 percentage points under President Bush I and by 8 percentage points under President Clinton, but it was

Chart 1.1 The Decline in Federal Tax Rates

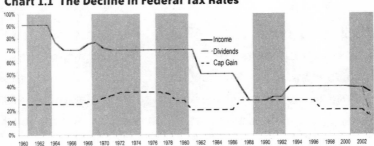

reduced to 35 percent in President Bush II's first term. In addition, the top rate of taxation on dividends and capital gains was reduced to 15 percent. The relatively prosperous period that followed was due, in large measure, to the efforts by Presidents Kennedy, Reagan, and Bush II to stimulate the economy with tax rate reductions. In fact, it is quite likely that an unsung hero of the expansion during the 1990s was the bipartisan 1986 Tax Reform Act.

The Nobel laureate Edward Prescott found an inverse correlation between tax rates and labor supply through his analysis of cross-country comparisons.[7] It is fascinating to see that many emerging economies are adopting low rates of taxation or a flat tax based on their observation that low rates help spur economic expansion.

President Bush II's tax cuts have been the subject of considerable debate. Structured to expire on certain dates unless Congress takes contrary action, these cuts still leave the top marginal tax rate 7 percentage points above the level bequeathed by President Reagan and his bipartisan majority, and loopholes and preferences have reappeared. These days it is rare to hear a political figure argue for the return of rates to pre-Reagan levels. On the contrary, most discussion focuses on keeping the rates low and simplifying the tax structure in the spirit of 1986. Certainly a key consideration in any debate on tax reform should be the potential impact on saving and investment, essential ingredients for a strong economic expansion.

The U.S. economy has also benefited from its flexibility, dynamism, and creativity. Flexibility, one of its most important attributes, is apparent in the movement of people into, out of, and within the labor force; in the creation and expiration of new businesses; and in the ebb and flow of the largest businesses. The late Joseph Schumpeter called capitalism a system of creative destruction, and this is nowhere more evident than in the flexibility of the U.S. economy.[8]

Examples of flexibility abound. For instance, the government reports the net number of jobs gained or lost each month. Usually the number is positive, reflecting the expansion of the economy. But that number obscures the reality of the high rate of job changes within the mix. The gross number of jobs gained and lost has ranged between six million and nine million per quarter over the past ten years.[9] For example, in 2005 just over twenty-nine million jobs were lost while more than thirty-one million were created.[10] The reported net figure of two million did not begin to describe the huge mobility within the American economy. This flexibility in the U.S. labor force is one explanation for the United States' ability to adapt so readily to new developments.

The large mobility in the labor force is likely to continue, and perhaps even increase, in the dynamic economy of the future. Therefore, it is clear that in any reform of the programs providing income for the elderly and access to health care for everyone, benefits should be associated with individuals rather than with institutions so that workers can change jobs without sacrificing important benefits.

The U.S. business picture is not only flexible but also dynamic. Over the last fifteen years, the number of new businesses created and the number that expired per year have ranged between five hundred thousand and six hundred thousand.[11] The net figure is usually positive, but the real point is the continuing impetus to develop new enterprises that help the U.S. economy maintain a competitive edge, since many grow and challenge existing companies.

Big businesses are subject to the same kind of competitive pressure. In May 1896 the Dow Industrial Average was made up of American Cotton Oil, American Sugar, American Tobacco, Chicago Gas, General Electric, Distilling & Cattle Feeding, Laclede Gas, National Lead, North American (a holding company), Tennessee Coal & Iron, U.S. Leather, and U.S. Rubber.[12] Only one, GE, is still recognizable. Of the companies listed in the Fortune 500 in 1960, quite a few were missing from the list by 1970, 1980, or 1990. For example, 306 of the companies listed in 1960 were no longer there in 1990. Even large companies are subject to mergers, acquisitions, and competitive pressures that can reduce their relative importance in the business world, and the United States is more willing than many other countries to encourage this kind of dynamism. Despite occasional relapses into a bailout mentality, as seen in the cases of Lockheed and Chrysler, the dominant theme is to allow competition, including foreign competition, to operate and cleanse the system of companies that have lost their competitive edge. Opportunities for new companies arise in large part because existing companies are permitted to fail. This is a prime illustration of Schumpeter's concept of creative destruction, and it is a powerful reason for the productivity of the U.S. economy and labor force.

This flexible and dynamic U.S. economy is also creative. Many of today's new industries did not exist thirty years ago. Consider the emergence of the cell phone, the widespread use of personal computers, the Internet, the hybrid car, satellite TV, digital cable, arthroscopic and laser surgery, and nanotechnology, among a multitude of other new developments. Research and development activity has thrived in the United States and many other countries throughout the post–World War II period. In 2002, for example, total R & D spending in the United States was about 2.6 percent of GDP, well above the level of spending by most Organization for Economic Cooperation and Development (OECD) countries. Patent activity is another important indicator of innovation, and patent applications, which have always been strong, have nearly tripled over the last ten to fifteen years. The number of patents issued shows a lag as the Patent

Office struggles to keep up with the flood of applications. Venture capital activity is still another gauge of innovation, and U.S. activity as a percentage of GDP is large compared with other countries. The United States invented venture capitalism, got a head start in it, and has never looked back. Once again, given the size of the U.S. economy, the total money devoted to venture investment in the United States dominates that of any other country.

International Trade and the Balance of Payments

The United States, in another largely positive development, has become more heavily involved in the international economic system throughout the post–World War II period. Wise statesmen at the end of that war reflected on the damage done to the global economy and international relations by the wave of protectionism that had swept the world in the 1920s and 1930s. They set out to design a different economic system that, through a series of negotiations, would gradually reduce tariff barriers and other impediments to trade. The negotiations succeeded brilliantly, and the world is now much more open and much more prosperous than a collection of relatively closed economies could ever be.

In the United States, exports and imports as a proportion of GDP have grown dramatically, and because the GDP is so large, that growth is even more stunning in

absolute numbers. Exports and imports together account
for almost one-fourth of U.S. economic output. The
United States is heavily involved in the world economy
and has benefited greatly from that involvement.

In the last twenty-five years there have been two
surges in imports relative to exports, leaving negative
balances of trade. By 2006 that deficit had reached more
than 6 percent of GDP but has since declined to less
than 5 percent of GDP.[13] A negative balance of trade is
not automatically good or bad. In fact, the numbers represent considerable benefits: Consumers have a wide
variety of products to choose from, prices are disciplined by international competition, and many overseas
markets are open for the export of U.S. products.

Some Problems

Although in many respects—stable prices and growth
rates, low tax rates, and dynamism—the U.S. economy
is as healthy as its citizens, there are problems on the
horizon. The U.S. rate of saving is by far the lowest of
any major country. Personal saving rates have fallen
dramatically and by now are essentially at zero. Back in
the 1980s the rate was in the 10 to 12 percent range, and
in the early 1990s it was still in the 7 to 8 percent range.
Certainly one part of the explanation is that the huge
boom in home values and asset prices more generally
during the past ten to fifteen years has resulted in a dramatic increase in household wealth. People may reason

that if their net worth is rising, saving out of their current income is unnecessary. If this is the case, the saving rate will likely rebound as housing prices have leveled off or even declined in many markets and as the rate of increase in other asset values moderates.

The federal deficit is of course an act of dissaving, even though it was running at the relatively low rate of 1.2 percent of GDP in fiscal year 2007. Nevertheless, if the private and public sector saving performances are added together, the result is that saving in the United States is not sufficient to finance this country's own investments. Fortunately the United States has an attractive investment climate with a relatively low risk/reward ratio. Thus savers in other countries are willing to invest in the United States, allowing the U.S. investment level to remain strong.

Adjustment problems must be faced in the United States and other countries as moderation of this large imbalance of saving and investment takes place. Beyond that, savers from other countries are, in a sense, sending us a message that should ring loud and clear in our ears: Those who save and invest own the assets and the income stream generated by those assets. If Americans saved more, their ownership of assets in the United States or elsewhere in the world economy would be greater and would enhance American claims on the U.S. and world economic pie. The impact on saving should be reflected in any consideration of policies to reform the entitlement programs.

Any examination of the U.S. economy must include the issue of immigration, which has always played an important role in American life. Over the course of its history and the ebb and flow of immigration waves, the United States has learned better than many other countries how to assimilate immigrants into its society. In turn, American culture has been modified and has benefited from the diverse talents and contributions of those who have come to its shores.

Today every country is struggling with the immigration issue. In this age of terror, the visa process requires special scrutiny. Ways must be developed to balance the desire to welcome those who can make a contribution with the need to prevent entrance by those who are a threat. This difficult problem must be dealt with effectively for many reasons, including the ability to attract new citizens who will help sustain the competitive edge of the United States.

The immigration dilemma poses a potentially debilitating problem for higher education. Throughout most of the post–World War II period, the United States has been the country of choice for people from all over the world who were seeking the best in college and especially graduate education. Recent visa rules, however, have prevented many talented foreign students from enrolling in American universities. Their absence underlines the fact that, in many of the demanding disciplines so central to future progress, the United States is unable to produce enough sufficiently qualified

Chart 1.2 Share of Income in Top Quintile Divided by Share of Incomes in Bottom Quintiles

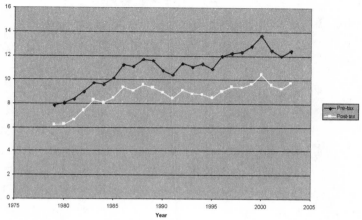

Source: Congressional Budget Office, Historical Effective Federal Tax Rates: 1979 to 2003, http://www.cbo.gov/ftpdoc.cfm?index=7000&type=1

Americans to fill the available openings. This problem stems from deficiencies in the K–12 curriculum and demands a concerted effort to improve the foundations of the U.S. education system.

Income distribution in the United States is yet another issue with relevance to entitlement programs. Chart 1.2 shows the ratio of the total income of the highest 20 percent of American households to the total income of the lowest 20 percent, both before and after taxes. Since after-tax income is what can be spent, let's concentrate on that.

The chart shows that the top 20 percent of households had just over six times as much after-tax income as the lowest 20 percent in the late 1970s. By the early 1980s, as the economy moved out of a period of inflationary trauma and as the performance of the stock market improved dramatically, the top 20 percent had gained a substantial advantage, and the ratio has hovered between eight and ten ever since. In the late 1990s this income ratio rose, and it remains at the high end of the range, meaning that on average, the top 20 percent of households have ten times as much after-tax income as the bottom 20 percent.

This picture of the distribution of income is moderated by the considerable movement of earners on the income distribution scale: High earners often drop to a lower level, and many low earners climb to a higher one. The picture is also moderated by the considerable impact of such programs as food stamps, welfare payments, and Medicaid that are directed to those with lower incomes. An important determinant of variations in income is the growing labor market premium for higher education and job market skills. The wages and salaries of those with college educations have dramatically outpaced the earnings of those with only high school educations or less. The country's goal should not be to reduce the income of the affluent but rather to increase the participation of lower-income households in the overall prosperity of the economy. Task number one in this regard is to improve the quality of K–12 education so that more workers are able to command more value in the job market.

Despite such problems, the U.S. economy is basically a great success story for clear underlying reasons. If these fundamental characteristics can be kept in good shape and if some of the associated problems can be addressed effectively, then the economy will continue to grow. The pie will become bigger and tastier and therefore easier to divide. Furthermore, this larger, expanding economy will play a crucial role in sustaining the success that is now producing longer, healthier lives and a higher standard of living for Americans.

CHAPTER TWO

The Iceberg Ahead

NOW FOR THE BAD NEWS. Promises to provide income for the elderly and health benefits for all Americans carry staggering prospective costs. These promises made by federal, state, and local governments and by private enterprises may generate costs that simply cannot be borne. The challenge is to find a way to fulfill the essence of these promises while reining in their future costs to manageable proportions. That is a tall order, and the process of reform has just begun. As Robert Frost put it in his "Stopping by Woods on a Snowy Evening":

> . . . I have promises to keep,
> And miles to go before I sleep . . .

Many well-informed, expert analysts have made projections of Social Security, Medicare, and Medicaid spending. All have come to essentially the same conclusions, even though many different forecasts can be generated by alternative assumptions. The message, in

Chart 2.1 Social Security, Medicare, and Medicaid Outlays as a Percentage of GDP, Fiscal Years 1950–2075

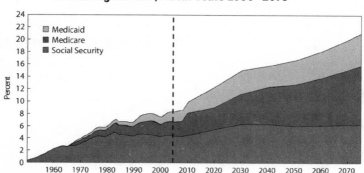

study after study, is that current programs will create costs that are unsustainable.

Economists Rudolph Penner and Eugene Steuerle, in "Budget Crisis at the Door," published estimates of entitlement costs in 2003.[1] Penner was the director of the Congressional Budget Office (CBO) and Steuerle was a high-level Treasury official, so they know what they are talking about. Their projections, shown in chart 2.1, reveal that federal spending on these programs, if they remain in their present form, will be in the range of 15 percent of the GDP twenty years from now and will represent more than 20 percent of GDP within seventy years. To put these estimates in perspective, the entire federal budget currently consumes about 20 percent of GDP.

This general picture is broadly confirmed by the 2007 annual reports of the Social Security and Medicare trustees and by projections using different assumptions made by the CBO, published in December 2005. These projections envision that:

1. Under the intermediate spending path, Medicare's costs would grow from 2.7 percent of GDP today to 8.6 percent in 2050. Total federal costs for Medicare and Medicaid combined would climb from 4.2 percent of GDP in 2005 to 12.6 percent in 2050.

2. The higher-spending path, in which the assumed rate of excess cost growth for health care of 2.5 percentage points is slightly *lower* than the long-term historical average, results in future costs that are seemingly unsustainable. Federal costs for Medicare and Medicaid as a percentage of GDP would nearly double—to 8.1 percent—in 2020 and reach 21.9 percent in 2050.[2]

The projections of the Social Security trustees are no more reassuring. In 2007 the board said that Social Security expenditures will exceed dedicated tax revenue in 2017.[3] They further said that the system's unfunded liability over a 75-year window is $4.7 trillion.[4]

John Goodman, the president of the National Center for Policy Analysis, in testimony before the House Ways and Means Committee in 2005, presented a similar outlook. He concluded:

> In just 15 years, the federal government will have to raise taxes, reduce other spending or borrow $761 billion to keep its promises to America's senior citizens. As the years pass, the size of the deficits will continue to grow. Without changes in worker payroll tax rates or senior citizen benefits, the shortfall

in Social Security and Medicare revenues compared to promised benefits will top more than $2 trillion in 2030, $4 trillion in 2040, and $7 trillion in 2050.[5]

The chorus of warnings continues. In his January 2007 testimony to the Senate Budget Committee, Chairman of the Federal Reserve Ben Bernanke stated, "The longer we wait, the more severe, the more draconian, the more difficult the adjustment is going to be."[6]

Recognition that the costs of entitlement programs are growing rapidly and are projected to eat up the entire federal budget is neither controversial nor new. In 1993, President Clinton created the Bipartisan Commission on Entitlement and Tax Reform. Chaired by Senator J. Robert Kerrey (Democrat from Nebraska) and Senator John Danforth (Republican from Missouri) and composed of members from both sides of the aisle, the commission projected that under 1994 law, entitlement spending in addition to the federal employee retirement system would consume the entire federal budget by 2030. Fortunately it appears that the commission's projection will not materialize quite so soon, but the growth rate has merely been trimmed, thereby postponing, but not diminishing, the fiscal crisis.

From 1946 to 2005, federal revenues averaged just under 18.1 percent of GDP and never exceeded 21 percent.[7] At the height of World War II, federal revenues as a percent of GDP were under 21 percent. In fact, the only other time federal revenues approached 21 percent of GDP was in the late years of the Clinton administration.[8] These numbers should make it clear that the fiscal imbalance created by the growth of the large federal entitlement programs is a problem that must be addressed by changing the structures of the programs. If Medicare, Medicaid, and Social Security were to grow as projected, they would require levels of taxation dramatically higher than any seen before. If the CBO's high-cost assumptions were to become reality, federal tax revenue as a percentage of GDP would have to double in order to produce a balanced budget. Of course such high tax rates would not be a solution. On the contrary, they would ruin the economy.

These spending projections call for sober consideration. They can be tweaked, and assumptions can be changed, but the result will always be spending far, far in excess of any precedent in U.S. history. The message is that changes are necessary, not optional, and there is an urgent need to put them into effect. For example, present payroll tax revenues, presumably dedicated to the Social Security system, will continue to outrun benefit payments for almost another decade, but this surplus is already starting to shrink and is being spent as though it were part of general revenues. The sooner these funds are used to cushion the change to a sustainable system, the easier the transition will be. And the sooner a sustainable system is in place, the more confidently potential beneficiaries can plan for their futures. Every year of delay is an opportunity lost.

State and City Promises

The all-too-real problem of funding pension promises made by both state and local governments is
broadly discernable, but the cost of health promises is
just now beginning to surface. The Government
Accounting Standards Board (GASB) has published
new rules governing accounting practices for health
benefits for retirees. These rules require state and
local governments to switch to accrual-based
accounting, in which the present value of promises
for the future must be publicly acknowledged, bringing pressure to show how these costs are to be
financed. This accounting method more accurately
reflects long-term liabilities, but local governments
have generally used pay-as-you-go accounting, meaning they acknowledge the costs only as they actually
pay the benefits. The result is that they mask their
future financial liabilities.

As the snow is cleared from Robert Frost's woods,
more promises that have simply staggering costs will be
revealed. The following examples hint at the serious-
ness of the problem.

Maryland, which until recently used pay-as-you-go
accounting, provides some of the most generous
health benefits in the nation to its retired state
employees. To comply with the new GASB rules, the
Maryland Department of Budget and Management
commissioned a study to calculate the magnitude of

its unfunded liability. The answer: $20 billion, or nearly double Maryland's annual general fund budget.[9] To prefund its liability over a thirty-year window, the state would have to contribute $1.9 billion each year, or approximately $340 per resident.

New Jersey is another state in deep trouble. As reported in the *New York Times* on July 25, 2007, unfunded promises of health care to New Jersey government retirees are now estimated to cost $58 billion, an amount nearly twice the size of the state's debt.[10]

The GASB rule change also led the Los Angeles Unified School District to commission a study that found an estimated $5 billion unfunded liability for retiree health care.[11] To fund this liability fully, the district would have to deposit $500 million, approximately 8 percent of the district's overall budget, into the bank each year for the next thirty years.

State and local governments have made generous promises of retirement benefits to their employees, but many of these governments have neither set aside funds to pay these benefits nor properly accounted for them. An extreme example of unrealistic promises is found in San Diego. Among the many mistakes it made, San Diego raised retirement benefits for city employees in 2002, underfunded the system, and hid what was going on. By 2005 the city had a full-blown scandal on its hands, with a $1.4 billion unfunded pension liability and, once retiree health benefits were factored in, more than \$2 billion in total liabilities.[12] The fallout from the scandal included the resignation of the mayor and a number of other top officials as well as a federal criminal probe.[13]

Promises are all too easy to make when the responsibility for paying them falls to someone else at some time in the distant future. New York City leads the pack in this practice. Its pension system is so generous that the pension accrual of city firefighters would require a contribution of an additional 60 percent of their pay. Unfortunately, New York has followed questionable actuarial assumptions and fooled itself into thinking it was completely solvent. Its chief actuary, Robert C. North, says the official numbers are "meaningless." He thinks that New York is approximately \$49 billion in the hole on its pension funds, an amount equal to the city's publicly disclosed outstanding debt.[14]

San Diego and New York may be the most egregious examples, but generous, underfunded government pension plans appear to be the norm. To put it simply, government employees want raises, and lawmakers want votes, but lawmakers do not want to pay salary increases out of the current year's budget. The solution? Raise pensions, the costs of which do not show up in pay-as-you-go accounting. Lawmakers—and not just those at the local and state levels—should not make promises that will have to be paid for by future generations. If they cannot fund the promises, they should not make them. Accrual accounting will help dramatize the importance of that rule.

So the cost to the *federal* government of entitlement programs is only part of the iceberg. In varying degrees, states match federal spending on Medicaid. Because they do not have the luxury of running deficits and because the costs of their entitlement promises are now rising, they are currently feeling the pain of a squeeze on budgets, with commensurate pressure on spending in other vital areas. For example, in 2003, twenty-one states spent more on Medicaid than on K–12 education.[15] States have also made large pension commitments to their employees, typically through defined benefit programs.[16] Funding for these programs is usually in place but is typically inadequate for the prospective costs. Many big cities and small towns also have pension and health care promises to keep.

Insuring Private Commitments

Private employers are confronted by many of the same problems that governments face. They too made promises in the form of defined benefit retirement systems and health programs that place heavy burdens on their current and future cash flows. Some of these promises will become obligations of the federal government. This is because the promises of private defined benefit pension plans are partially backed by the federal government's Pension Benefit Guaranty Corporation (PBGC). The PBGC collects premiums from private companies and partially insures their pension plans. Insurance payments to the PBGC have not kept pace with pension plan defaults as companies in bankruptcy, such as United Airlines, have turned their programs and the inadequate funding for them over to the government's guaranty system, which is now woefully underfunded.

In many ways, the corporate health care picture is even more out of control than its pension system. Companies have made promises based on their predicted ability to fund them in the future. However, older companies, in particular, now have large numbers of retirees, and the unfunded costs of their pension and health care systems are crippling, especially in a globally competitive environment. Before the recent buyout of their obligations, it is estimated that General Motors' health care commitments to its retirees cost the company $1,500 per car.[17] GM faces vigorous competition from such companies as Toyota and Honda, which have no comparable cost overhang.

Pulling private and government programs together, we see that health care spending in the United States has risen dramatically, from 5.2 percent of GDP in 1960 to 16 percent by 2006, and is expected to reach 18.7 percent of GDP by 2014.[18] The portion of these expenditures paid for by the federal government has increased steadily from 11.3 percent in 1965 to 34 percent in

2006.[19] In addition, the federal and state governments lost approximately $200 billion in revenue in 2006 because of their failure to classify health insurance premiums as taxable income.[20]

Clearly the choice is not between taking action and maintaining the status quo. Change is necessary. The urgent question is how to implement changes that will bring costs under control while providing income for the elderly and a comprehensive, high-quality health care system.

CHAPTER THREE

Age and the
Labor Force

THE PROSPECTS FOR SUCCESS in dealing with specific reforms of Social Security and health care programs will be significantly enhanced by encouraging greater participation in the labor force and an increase in the size of the economy.

Thinking of the economy as a pie, we can clearly see that the larger the pie, the easier it will be to allocate money to entitlement spending. This highlights the importance of making the pie as big as possible. Call this the pie test for judging proposals for reform. Proposals that increase participation in the labor force, particularly by older workers, pass the pie test with flying colors.

The mounting financial difficulties of Social Security stem from a long history of increasing benefit levels when revenues from the payroll tax far exceeded benefit flows and from the continuing trend of increased longevity. As Americans live longer, they spend more years out of the workforce. In fact, over the past seventy years all the extra average adult lifetime has been spent in retirement. To the extent that this represents a free choice between the benefits of leisure as compared with the benefits of work, who can complain? As we become more affluent, we spend more of our resources on leisure. The fact is, however, that many aspects of the system discourage the choice of work as an individual grows older.

In 1965 the typical male worker exited the labor force at approximately age sixty-six, but by 2003 he was retiring three years earlier. In addition, the typical male worker who retired in 1965 at age sixty-six could expect to live an additional thirteen years. But by 2003, when the typical male retired at age sixty-three, his life expectancy had increased to almost nineteen years. Not only were men retiring earlier, but they were also living longer, healthier lives. The result is that the average length of retirement for men has grown by almost 50 percent since 1965, with about half the increase attributable to improved longevity and the other half to earlier retirement.

There are a variety of ways to estimate the possible impact on the economy of a change in current patterns of labor force participation. If, in 2003, men in the fifty to seventy-four age bracket had the labor force participation rates of men in 1965, there would have been approximately 2.8 million more workers, or 2 percent of the labor force. That increase would affect the GDP year after year.

Remember some important developments. The conventional method of measuring age, years since birth, fails to adjust to rapidly improving life expectancy. It makes no sense to use the same age categories for the elderly in the twenty-first century that were used in the nineteenth and twentieth centuries. Given our rapidly improving life expectancy, a better measure of age is mortality risk, or the chance of dying within a year, which mounts naturally with increases in age to levels known as mortality milestones. A person with a high mortality risk is old, one with a low mortality risk is young, and two people with the same mortality risk are, in this way of looking at it, effectively the same age.

Examination of the evolution of these milestones over the past sixty years reveals that the age at which various mortality milestones are reached has risen considerably for both men and women in the United States. For example, a seventy-eight-year-old woman in 2000 had the same mortality risk as a sixty-nine-year-old woman in 1940 (4 percent), so they may be thought of as the same age, while sixty-five-year-old men in 2000 faced the same mortality risk as did fifty-nine-year-old men in 1970 (2 percent).[1] In 2000 seventy-year-old women also faced a 2 percent mortality risk. In a very real sense, sixty-five-year-old men in 2000, fifty-nine-year-old men in 1970, and seventy-year-old women in 2000 are the same age in the sense that they share the same mortality risk.

This way of thinking changes everything, including the number of elderly, the amount that should be saved

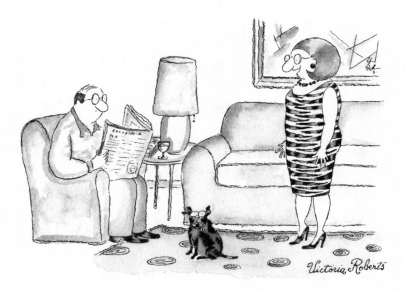

"Good news honey—seventy is the new fifty."

for retirement, and the number of years an individual should consider working.

To take a different approach, think of workers in their twenties today who will retire around 2050, and consider two possibilities: (1) They will retire at the same ages as today's retirees, or (2) when they retire, they will enjoy the same length of retirement as today's retirees. If the length of retirement were stabilized, then the number of labor hours worked in 2050 would be at least 9 percent greater than under the first scenario. This alone would result in a 6 to 7 percent larger GDP. If the extra labor were matched by a larger capital stock, then the GDP would be at least 9 percent greater. This translates to more than $1 trillion in today's economy, a hefty increase in the size of the pie that would allow much more room for maneuvering in entitlement reform. That leeway will surely be needed because no matter what reforms are adopted, spending on health care and income support is bound to rise as the U.S. population ages.

One reason we want to expand labor force participation is that Medicare, Medicaid, and Social Security can be expected to cost substantially more in the future simply because of the increasing numbers of people to be covered. As a society we have a limited set of choices to make about these programs and how to finance them.

Consider, for example, an upper-middle-class family of four with an $80,000 annual after-tax income. The first time we meet this family, we note two facts. First, they have no health insurance, and second, one of the children has a potentially fatal disease that is untreatable. The latter fact, though tragic, does not present a financial problem because the illness is truly untreatable.

The next time we meet this family, their luck has changed. An effective treatment has been developed for the child, but at $1,500 per month, it is expensive. The family celebrates the good news but then sobers up in the face of the new financial reality. They have only three choices: (1) They could forgo the new medication on the ground that they cannot afford it (a decision no parent is likely to make); (2) they could significantly restructure their lifestyle and reduce their spending on everything else by $18,000 per year; or (3) the parents could take on additional jobs, working in the evenings or on weekends, increase their total income by $18,000, and approximately maintain their standard of living. Most people would probably choose a combination of the last two options, with working harder being an important part of the solution.

The U.S. economy itself faces a similar problem. The biotech revolution will produce many effective, but costly, medications, some of which will alleviate currently untreatable diseases. As a society we shall have three basic options. First, we could decide not to use the new technologies because they are too expensive, an unlikely, and undesirable, choice. That leaves the other two options: squeezing out funding for all these medical treatments by reducing the amount of money spent on everything else, or choosing to work harder and enjoy the new medical technologies as well as a higher standard of living. For the economy as a whole, working harder translates into working more years and retiring later. With longer life expectancies, retiring later does not mean shorter retirements. All in all, postponing retirement is a natural and desirable choice given the huge health care and retirement costs facing the nation.

This chapter is designed to make a simple point: A rise in labor force participation will ease considerably the problems of dealing effectively with growing entitlement costs. Obviously people cannot be ordered to work longer; they value leisure and make trade-offs between the income from additional work and more time for themselves. Obviously the trade-offs will be influenced by the proportion of extra income that remains after taxes have been paid. In making these decisions, however, they will be affected by a structure of rewards and penalties. The trouble is that many disincentives for older people to work have been built into our systems along with disincentives for employers to hire older workers. If the incentive structure is changed, people will respond.

One misunderstanding we ought to dispel immediately is the so-called lump of labor hypothesis. This philosophy maintains that there is a fixed amount of work to be done—a lump of labor—so if the elderly can be encouraged to leave the workforce, there will be more jobs for the young. This zero-sum thinking is simply wrong. Economists treat labor as one of the primary inputs into economic output, and the more input, the more output. Nonetheless, the lump of labor hypothesis has widespread popular appeal, and numerous policies have been based on it, particularly in Europe. To a degree, the U.S. Social Security system was developed with this idea in mind: The expectation was that benefits would induce older workers to leave the labor force. By and large, however, policies designed to create opportunities for the young by encouraging older workers to retire have been colossal failures. The same European countries that implemented early retirement programs have long suffered from chronically high youth unemployment.

The United States has a number of policies that, intentionally or unintentionally, are consistent with the discredited lump of labor concept. These policies, which tend to discriminate against older workers or those with very long careers, should be eliminated. Americans who wish to work for more than forty years, into their sixties, seventies, or eighties, should not be penalized with high tax rates. On the contrary, they should be rewarded. By working longer, they help themselves as well as everyone else by increasing the size of the economic pie. Here are some steps that would level the playing field for those who want to pursue long careers.

Proposals to Increase Labor Force Participation by Older Americans

1. Establish a category of paid-up workers who are exempt from payroll taxes after they have worked a full career.

Allow workers to stop contributing payroll taxes once they have largely stopped accruing benefits. In terms of current law, this would take effect after thirty-five years of work, but this could be revised to forty years (and indexed to increases in life expectancy) if the next proposal were adopted. The paid-up concept is common in private insurance policies, and its adoption would have a dramatic effect on incentives for older workers to remain in the labor force and for employers to hire older workers. The worker would take home more of his or her income because there would no longer be a 6.2 percent deduction from his or her earnings for the Social Security tax. The employer would benefit from hiring older workers because there would be no 6.2 percent tax to pay on their behalf. Today a very small percentage of Social Security's revenue comes from individuals who have worked more than forty years. Change in this policy would be revenue neutral for the government as a whole with only a moderate response in terms of a longer time at work, since added income tax payments would likely make up for the lost revenue.

2. Use forty years of earnings, rather than thirty-five, in the calculation of Social Security benefits.

Social Security benefits are currently calculated using the average of the highest thirty-five years of annual earnings.[2] This means that while the thirty-third, thirty-fourth, and thirty-fifth years of working are noticeably increasing the Social Security benefits an individual will receive in retirement, the thirty-sixth, thirty-seventh, and subsequent years of earnings may or may not enter the calculation of benefits. If they do, they increase benefits only to the extent that they replace a lower year of earnings from earlier in the worker's career. Therefore, the incentive to work beyond thirty-five years is much lower than for the first thirty-five years. In particular, part-time work after a career of thirty-five or more years will usually have no effect on a worker's Social Security benefits, making the Social Security contributions paid in those years a pure tax on working.

One way to alleviate this problem is to count the highest forty years of annual earnings instead of the highest thirty-five. This would send the message that forty, instead of thirty-five, years of earnings constitute a full career, a point that a significant number of men and women hit as early as age fifty-two. The definition of a full career probably should be indexed to increase as life expectancy increases so that it would grow gradually to forty-one years, then forty-two years, and so on.

This change, done in isolation, would constitute a benefit reduction because the average of a worker's highest forty years of earnings is in most cases less than the average of that same worker's highest thirty-five years of earnings. On an aggregate basis, Social Security would be paying approximately 7 percent less in benefits if this policy were instituted alone. To make up for this reduction, all benefits could be increased by 7 percent so that the policy would be benefit neutral overall. There would be some winners from this policy change—namely, individuals who work longer careers—whereas individuals with shorter careers would fare worse. However, the incentives to continue working beyond thirty-five years would be greatly improved.

3. Allow each year of actual earnings to count the same in the Social Security benefit calculation.

Social Security discourages long careers because its system, which is designed to help low-income Americans, winds up helping high-income workers who have short careers. An individual who earns just above the minimum wage over the span of a long career will be correctly identified by the Social Security system as having low lifetime earnings. However, an individual with relatively higher earnings per year over a short career span would also qualify as a low average earner by Social Security calculations. This inconsistency occurs because Social Security figures out average earnings on the basis of the highest thirty-five years of earnings, which would include zeros for those years in which an individual had no earnings. The system then incorrectly treats that person as a lifetime low-income earner. As a result, extending one's career from fifteen to twenty years raises the calculated benefit more than extending it from thirty to thirty-five years. Later years of work count less toward Social Security benefits than early years.

We propose changing the method of calculating Social Security benefits to allow each year of work to count the same. This would involve calculating an individual's average earnings exclusively on the basis of years worked to indicate more accurately whether such a worker is a low- or high-income earner. This amount would be used to determine the monthly retirement benefit the worker would be eligible to receive if he or she worked a full career. The resulting benefit amount would then be prorated on the basis of the number of years worked. For example, a worker with a ten-year career would receive half as much as he would have from working a twenty-year career. This would give the worker the same incentive to work the second set of ten years as the first, unlike the current system, in which later years of work count less than earlier years in terms of earning future Social Security benefits

This policy, similar to the earlier proposals, can be enacted in a way that is, overall, neutral to Social Security finances. Individuals who work shorter careers would fare worse, but individuals who work longer careers would fare better, and there would be a larger incentive to work a long career.

4. Eliminate the high marginal tax rates faced by Social Security beneficiaries who receive outside income.

If an individual has very little or no outside income, none of his or her Social Security benefits are taxable. But if an individual's income combined with half of his or her yearly Social Security benefits exceeds $25,000, a portion of his or her Social Security benefits becomes taxable. This portion could be as much as 85 percent. The $25,000 floor was established in 1986 and has never been adjusted for inflation.

What is the result of this tax treatment? Imagine a sixty-five-year-old individual in a 25 percent income tax bracket. This worker turns sixty-six and decides to take Social Security. If he continues working, what would his marginal income tax rate be? The obvious guess would be 25 percent, but that would be wrong. The correct answer could be as high as 46 percent because as an individual earns more income, more of his or her Social Security benefits become taxable. During a second tax phase-in period, $1.00 of outside income causes $0.85 of Social Security benefits to become taxable. Therefore, $1.00 of outside income triggers not $0.25, but $0.46, in income tax (25 percent of $1.85).

Viewed properly, these figures represent taxes on income, not Social Security benefits. It is the magnitude of other taxable income (labor earnings, dividends, interest, and so on) that triggers the taxability of Social Security. The step at which an extra $1.00 of taxable income makes an additional $0.85 of Social Security benefits taxable should be eliminated so that those who work while receiving Social Security are not so heavily penalized with high tax rates.[3]

5. Examine the relationship between eligibility for Medicare and eligibility for health benefits under a corporate plan.

Under the current system, someone working for an employer that offers health insurance loses much of his or her Medicare eligibility; the private plan is the primary payer and Medicare becomes the secondary payer. For many, this amounts to a tax on work because the employer's contribution to the health insurance plan reduces compensation to the worker. Indeed, one reason for the recent lag in wage rates is the diversion of more compensation into various benefits. We propose that once individuals reach the age of sixty-five and become eligible for Medicare, they should receive it whether or not they work. Then employers would be relieved of the costs of health insurance for their Medicare-eligible workers. Such a shift would make work more attractive to older employees and the hiring of older workers much more attractive to employers.

6. Remove the notch that Medicaid beneficiaries face when deciding whether to work.

Medicaid, government-provided health insurance for the poor financed jointly by the federal government and the states, varies somewhat across state boundaries. But in every case, eligibility for Medicaid involves an income or wealth test. A family is either eligible or ineligible for Medicaid. If its income increases above the eligibility threshold, it loses Medicaid—not just a portion, but all of it. An extra $100 of earnings could cause the family to lose health insurance worth thousands of dollars. Economists call this trigger effect of extra income a "notch," but most people would call it a cliff: If the family crosses the income eligibility threshold, they have just driven over a precipice. The effect on that family's situation can be disastrous.

Research on the welfare system has increased awareness of this notch problem and the importance of solving it so that low-income individuals are encouraged to work through the notch levels. A way to accomplish this result will be presented in chapter 10.

As we have noted, the U.S. population is aging and the Social Security and health care plans now in place will generate costs that cannot be sustained. The programs must be reformed. But even before reforms are put in place, a preliminary set of actions can spur positive change in both areas. The larger the rate of participation in the labor force, the larger the gross national product (GNP). This is the pie that will be shared, and the larger it is, the easier is the sharing process.

We have identified a variety of ways in which the present systems could be altered. If these ideas are adopted, participation in the labor force will rise, particularly by those in the older age-groups. The results: more income for elderly workers and a bigger national product. These changes will pass the pie test!

PART TWO

Social Security

CHAPTER FOUR

Income for
Retirement

ONE OF LIFE'S BIGGEST decisions is when to leave the labor force and enter retirement. The traditional age for this transition has been sixty-five. But in the past few decades the underlying factors have changed dramatically. People are healthier, wealthier, and living longer. Many leave the labor force before they turn sixty-five.

These facts highlight the importance of the sources, adequacy, and dependability of retirement income on decisions about when to retire. Social Security will be a special focus of our attention later in this chapter and in subsequent chapters, but the elderly also have income from their own resources and from employment-based pension programs of various kinds. Like the Social Security system, these programs are under strain, and they are changing. These developments are important in their own right, but because they are key components of retirement income, they also bear on what should be done about the problem of Social Security.

During the Great Depression of the 1930s, central

preoccupations about the economy obviously included not only the high unemployment levels of the time but also the lack of income by many Americans who could no longer work. The Social Security system has its roots in this era. It was developed partly as a way to take older people out of the labor force to make jobs for younger workers and partly as a system to provide income for people over sixty-five years of age.

Similarly, pension programs for the employees of state and local governments and of private employers got started at this time and became common as the post–World War II years moved along. As noted in chapter 2, all these promises to pay employees a flow of defined benefits in their retirement years have created a large part of the iceberg ahead.

The federal government, with its ability to run substantial deficits year after year, can, even if unwisely, kick the Social Security can a little farther down the road, but many others are unable to do so. State and local governments, many private entities, and governments of some other countries have no such alternative. They are already working on this issue.

In Japan and many Western European countries, where the demographic weight of older populations is already powerful and growing rapidly, the problem must be addressed. Similarly, the pension programs of many states and cities in the United States are far more generous than the capacity of those units of government to finance them. Usually their pension promises are supported by dedicated funds, but generous benefits and unanticipated longevity have made these funds inadequate. Because state and city governments have to balance their budgets, they are forced to confront the problem.

Private employers are also feeling the weight of pension program costs because they operate in private markets and are up against global competitors that often do not have these costs to carry. They, too, seek alternatives.

The structure of the pension issue is the same everywhere and stems from two inexorable realities related to the shifting demographics of the population: (1) An increasing proportion of individuals are of benefit-receiving age and a decreasing proportion of people are of paying-in age, and (2) there is every prospect that longevity will continue to increase. These developments were typically not anticipated when retirement plans were first established.

Defined benefit pension systems have historically been similar at the federal, state, and private-sector levels. They promise a specific amount of money every year for life, usually beginning at age sixty-five, but many systems have incentives that encourage retirement at even earlier ages. It is easy to see how this structure leads to inevitable problems; the system is financed on the basis of paying current costs out of current revenues while simply ignoring the rapidly mounting costs of commitments to be paid for in future years, the pay-as-you-go system. The

problem exists even in cases in which funds were established for investments on behalf of future benefit obligations because current longevity trends were not taken
into account in the funding assumptions.

Private employers in the United States face growing
pressure to meet their commitments and restructure
the plans they offer their employees. A brief summary
of this developing problem will give a sense of the kinds
of solutions that may emerge in response to this pressure. The experiences of other countries as well as those
of private American employers will be instructive.

Private Employers

The structure of pension plans provided by private
employers has changed markedly over the last quarter
century, and the pace of change has accelerated in recent
years. Most new companies have adopted defined contribution (DC) plans instead of traditional defined benefit (DB) plans, and some older firms have switched to
defined contribution programs. DC plans include the
401(k) plans of private employers, 403(b) plans of nonprofit organizations, and 457 plans for government
employers. All defined contribution plans are character-
ized by a tax-deferred retirement account established by
the employer, who promises some formula of employer
contribution to it. Some employers offer to match
employee contributions. There are no promised retirement benefits. The retirement proceeds will be whatever

can be financed by the contributions and their investment returns. The participants bear whatever risks are inherent in the underlying investments. Nevertheless, defined contribution plans are popular with both employers and employees. Employers like their simplicity and the fact that the costs are known. Employees like the portability inherent in the plans. Even if they change jobs, they keep their accounts, including the employer contributions, provided that they have stayed with the employer longer than the vesting period.

DB plans, on the other hand, provide participants with a retirement benefit that is determined by a formula and paid for life. The formula varies from employer to employer, but it generally depends on the employee's age, salary, and number of years of service with the firm. For example, a company may promise its employees an annual benefit equal to 2 percent of their final year's salaries multiplied by their years of service once they have attained normal retirement age, as defined by the plan. An individual who works at this firm for thirty-two years will therefore receive 64 percent of his or her final year's salary from the pension plan at the plan's normal retirement age. The benefit amount may be reduced if the participant retires earlier to account for the fact that he or she is expected to receive benefits for a longer time. However, benefits are rarely augmented for later retirement. Thus, these individuals are often penalized for working beyond the normal retirement age. Employees are typically not required to make contributions into the plan's fund, nor do they make investment decisions; the employer bears the risks associated with funding the plan. Unlike DC plans, DB plans are not portable across firms. A participant who leaves his or her employer before five years of service may not receive any benefits from the pension plan.

The change in the relative importance of defined benefit and defined contribution plans is nothing short of remarkable. The number of defined contribution plans has always well exceeded defined benefit plans, inasmuch as that was the only reasonable approach for small employers. But when it comes to covered participants, the picture is sharply different.

In 1975, there were almost 2.4 times more participants in active defined benefit plans than in active defined contribution plans.[1] The numbers became about the same by 1985, but by 2002 the number of participants in defined benefit plans had diminished to about 40 percent of those in defined contribution plans. By now, in other words, the situation has totally reversed, with participants in defined contribution plans outnumbering those in defined benefit plans by 2.4 to 1.

This movement toward defined contribution plans has continued in recent years because of the growing costs of complying with defined benefit plan regulations and the uncertainty of those costs created by fluctuating markets and increasing longevity. In some cases, companies have gone bankrupt and their defined benefit plans have wound up in the hands of the Pension Benefit Guaranty Corporation (PBGC), the government agency that insures those plans. The PBGC is financed by required insurance premiums from defined benefit plans, but as defaults have risen, the revenue from the premiums has not been sufficient to offset the costs. In a recent spectacular case, United Airlines defaulted on its pension obligations when it declared bankruptcy and handed its inadequate pension assets and underfunded liabilities over to the PBGC. Because the maximum benefit guaranteed is $45,000 per year for those who retire at age sixty-five, some United employees took a beating. For example, United pilots with pensions over $100,000 per year received pension cuts of 50 to 75 percent. After the airline emerged from bankruptcy, it offered its employees a 401(k) defined contribution plan.

Although United Airlines had the biggest pension default in the history of the United States, its case is not particularly unusual. The PBGC has taken over the pension liabilities of US Airways, Bethlehem Steel, and Huffy Bicycles, to name just a few. Between 2002 and 2005, more than twenty companies defaulted on pension plans of more than $100 million in size. An even greater number of plans are underfunded; that is, their liabilities exceed their assets. Moreover, the PBGC itself is in trouble; in September 2004 the CBO estimated that its costs will exceed its premiums by $141.9 billion over the next twenty years.[2] Current law limits PBGC payouts to the assets it controls plus premiums. If projections become reality, individuals receiving pensions controlled by the PBGC will face another round of benefit cuts. The alternative is a bailout from the taxpayers.

The 2006 pension reform bill attempted to address the funding shortfalls of some corporate defined benefit pension plans and of the PBGC itself. By some estimates, the bill reduced the PBGC's unfunded liability by about one-third by raising the premiums that companies offering defined benefit plans pay to the PBGC and by imposing stricter funding standards for the plans. The added premiums and regulations likely make DB plans even less attractive than before to corporations. There is every reason to believe that the movement away from defined benefit plans and toward 401(k) offerings will continue and even accelerate.

Beyond private employers who are in financial trouble, perfectly healthy companies are also reviewing their posture on benefits. IBM, a robust company, has frozen its defined benefit plan and switched all future provisions for retirement to defined contribution plans. IBM will automatically deposit from 1 to 4 percent of an employee's pay into his or her 401(k) account and match dollar for dollar up to 6 percent of salary deferrals. Verizon has also switched to a defined contribution plan and will match employee contributions up to 6 percent of an employee's salary.

Evidently, private employers are reacting to pressures on their retirement systems by moving to defined con-

For information about permission to reproduce
selections from this book, write to Permissions,
W. W. Norton & Company, Inc.,
500 Fifth Avenue, New York, NY 10110

For information about special discounts for bulk
purchases, please contact W. W. Norton Special Sales at
specialsales@wwnorton.com or 800-233-4830

Manufacturing by RR Donnelley, Haddon
Book design by Charlotte Staub
Production manager: Anna Oler

Library of Congress Cataloging-in-Publication Data

Shultz, George Pratt, 1920–
Putting our house in order : a guide to social security and health
care reform / George P. Shultz and John B. Shoven ; with Matthew
Gunn and Gopi Shah Goda. — 1st ed.
p. cm.
Includes bibliographical references and index.
ISBN 978-0-393-06602-9 (hbk.)
1. Social security—United States—Management. 2. Health care
reform—United States. I. Shoven, John B. II. Title.
HD7125.S537 2008
362.1'04250973—dc22

                                                              2008001783

W. W. Norton & Company, Inc.
500 Fifth Avenue, New York, N.Y. 10110
www.wwnorton.com

W. W. Norton & Company Ltd.
Castle House, 75/76 Wells Street, London W1T 3QT

1 2 3 4 5 6 7 8 9 0

Putting Our House in Order

A Guide to Social Security and Health Care Reform

George P. Shultz AND
John B. Shoven *with*
Matthew Gunn AND
Gopi Shah Goda

W. W. NORTON & COMPANY
New York · London

tribution plans, the costs of which can be predicted. But how are employees affected by these shifts? Some argue that this development transfers risks from employers to employees, whose eventual benefits will reflect the uncertain returns of the financial marketplace. There is another side to this coin, however. As the preceding discussion shows, there are plenty of risks in defined benefit plans. Furthermore, employees gain a significant measure of protection because defined contribution plans create an asset that belongs to them. In the case of defined benefit plans, employees who change employers lose financially, but those with defined contribution plans take their accounts with them. Furthermore, if sizable contributions are made over an extended period of time and are prudently invested according to an age-related allocation of assets, experience shows there is a high probability that sufficient money will be available for retirement.

Pressure on the defined benefit plans provided by private employers has yielded a clear result: The defined contribution plan is the wave of the future. What is the federal government's role in this shift? Money put into a defined benefit plan by an employer is a deductible expense for the employer and is not taxable income for the employee. The employee eventually pays taxes, presumably in a lower tax bracket, on the income from the pension plan at retirement. The counterpart in the case of defined contributions is, in effect, a choice. Employees can put pretax dollars into their 401(k) plans, which contain employer and employee contributions, and pay tax on the money taken out. Alternatively, an employee can use Roth IRAs and Roth 401(k)s as savings vehicles. For these types of plans, individuals pay tax on the money they put in, but withdrawals are tax free.

One feature that has been lost in the switch away from defined benefit plans to defined contribution employment-based pensions is automatic enrollment. Under the old defined benefit plans, employees were automatically enrolled, so participation was 100 percent of those eligible. By contrast, defined contribution plans usually require employees to sign up for a 401(k) plan or its equivalent in order to participate. Employer-sponsored retirement plans have attractive tax features and frequently offer employer matching of employee contributions, an important benefit. But encouragement to enroll is uneven across employers, and follow-through by workers is much lower than might be preferred or expected. There is ample evidence that outcomes are different if employees must opt out of, rather than sign up for, participation. Researchers Brigitte Madrian and Dennis Shea found that in a private firm that switched its new employees to automatic enrollment in its 401(k) plan, participation increased from roughly 40 percent to more than 80 percent although no other changes had been made in the plan's characteristics.[3] This dramatic increase can be attributed both to participant inertia and to employees' acceptance of implicit investment advice from their employers. Clearly, given the tax advantages of this form of saving for retirement, enrollment in such a plan is a good deal for the vast majority of employees. Companies should be encouraged to make participation automatic unless employees actively choose to opt out, a step that would ensure much higher participation rates.

Particularly as automatic enrollment becomes universal among employers that offer defined contribution pension plans, the composition of the investment portfolio should be examined. Many employees will end up with what is called the default portfolio, into which the company puts the assets of those employees who do not make an active choice of investments. Ideally, default portfolios should be composed of a so-called life cycle fund (a balance of indexed stock and bond funds that is adjusted according to the age of the participant) or a broadly diversified equity portfolio. Neither money market funds nor the employer's stock should be designated as the default choice; these investments are inappropriate for most retirement savers. Firms that automatically put participants into money market funds have found, twenty years later, that some of those employees never changed their asset allocations. Money market funds have a role to play in the financial universe, but being a retirement accumulation vehicle is not one of them. Long-haul investments that are broadly diversified or indexed portfolios of stocks and bonds have a track record of superior returns over the long run.

Evidence of investor inertia is so strong that it could be used in other ways so as to institute a set of policies that encourage saving in this country. For instance, tax refunds could be invested in individual retirement accounts (IRAs) unless a taxpayer instructs otherwise. Also, employers could be encouraged to offer systematic saving plans over and above their pension plans through payroll deduction into tax-deferred accounts. Evidence shows that people usually do what is easy and automatic, and that is how saving plans should be offered.

In summary, private companies, always conscious of the bottom line, face mounting competitive pressure, in many cases on a global basis, and they have been among the first to act. Aware of the pressing need to balance their budgets, states and cities are also stirring. The federal government must follow.

Social Security

The Social Security system has been in effect now for almost three-quarters of a century. It operates as a pay-as-you-go system; the payroll taxes it collects from today's workers are used to pay benefits to today's beneficiaries. The original idea was that the benefits an individual received would reflect the contributions he or she made, as in an insurance policy. This relationship holds even though a degree of progressivity has always been present. Over most of its history, Social Security's revenues from payroll taxes have exceeded the actual benefits it has paid out. But instead of using these extra funds to back promises of future benefits, the government has used the money to make benefits increasingly generous or has simply spent the money as though it were part of general revenues. All attempts to fund future promises have failed. At this point it is widely acknowledged that the income stream generated by what is now a 12.4 percent payroll tax will start falling short of the benefits to be paid out by the time another decade passes. Compellingly, the gap between revenues and benefits has begun to narrow sharply, so the budget squeeze is now upon us.

The Social Security trust fund contains the surpluses, invested in government bonds, that have been generated by the system since its inception. One purpose of this trust fund is to help pay for future benefits. However, it will not be of much help for the eventual solvency of Social Security because the money that Social Security has transferred to the Treasury has not been saved but rather used to pay the day-to-day expenses of running the government. The bond purchases have built up to a bundle of federal government IOUs. In testimony before the 1994–1996 Social Security Advisory Board, Barry Bosworth of the Brookings Institution said that policy makers had been "playing games" with the money. He used the analogy of a family that saved for future college expenses by setting up a special savings fund. Each year they made the appropriate deposits into the fund, but during the year they kept borrowing from the fund and replacing the money with IOUs. By the time the children were of college age, the only thing in the college savings fund was a pile of IOUs.

Since the 1983 Greenspan Commission reform of Social Security, the Social Security Administration has been transferring its excess funds to the rest of the federal government. Apparently not a penny has been saved. A decade from now, these excesses may look like an accumulation of $4 trillion in bonds. The problem is that the federal government will have spent the money on other programs. The pile of IOUs will no more finance the retirement of the baby boomers than would the stock of college savings IOUs help the family just described send their children to college.

The inability of the trust fund to provide relief to future generations has been known for a long time. In 1937, Senator Arthur Vandenberg said:

> What has happened, in plain language, is that the pay-roll taxes for this branch of Social Security have been used to ease the contemporary burden of the general public debt or to render painless another billion of current Government spending, while the old-age pension fund gets a promise-to-pay which another generation of our grandsons and granddaughters can wrestle with, decades hence. It is one of the slickest arrangements ever invented. It fits particularly well into the scheme of things when the Federal Government is on a perpetual spending spree.[4]

More than sixty years later, in 1998, Senator Bob Kerrey testified: "We are not prefunding! The idea in 1983 was that we would prefund the baby boomers. We began to use it immediately for the expenditures of the general government. We didn't prefund anything."

The picture is clear. One government program, Social Security, has tried to save for and prefund the retirement of the baby boomers. Congress and the executive branch have spent it all. No saving has taken place, and all we are accumulating is a pile of IOUs. This situation must change, and the introduction of individual accounts is an appealing alternative. Participants would be allowed to own and control some part of their Social Security assets by channeling their contributions into individually owned invest-ment accounts. If surplus Social Security income were put into individual accounts and invested in indexed stock and bond funds, then other government pro-grams would have to get by without Congress's put-ting its hands into the Social Security cookie jar. The country's saving rate would be higher and future gen-erations of Americans would be better off.

The system's financial problem can look somewhat better or worse according to the assumptions that are made about prospective increases in longevity, but the basic problem remains: If the current payroll tax rate remains unchanged and if the system is to be solvent in the long run, changes in the benefit structure must be made. The current surplus of revenues over benefits, which is predicted to continue for about a decade, provides a cushion for transition costs, but that cushion is more like an hourglass: The longer you wait to use it, the less remains to be used.

Under these circumstances, you would think that the federal government would be energized to work on the problem, but this is hardly the case. Presidents Bill Clinton and George W. Bush have agreed, to a remarkable degree, on the need to do something and on the advantage of doing it sooner rather than later. Here is what one of them said to a group of Georgetown University undergraduates:

> This fiscal crisis in Social Security affects every generation. . . . It's very important that you understand this. . . . If you don't do anything, one of two things will happen—either it [Social Security] will go broke and you won't ever get it; or if we wait too long to fix it, the burden on society of taking care of our [the baby boom] generation's Social Security obligations will lower your income and lower your ability to take care of your children to a degree that most of us who are your parents think would be horribly wrong and unfair to you and unfair to the future prospects of the United States.

He went on to say, "Today, we're actually taking in a lot more money from Social Security taxes enacted in 1983 than we're spending out. Because we've run deficits, none of that money has been saved for Social Security." Finally, he warned that if nothing is done until the trust fund runs out of money, the choice will be "a huge tax increase in the payroll tax, or just about a 25 percent cut in Social Security benefits."[5]

Which president was this? It was President Clinton in a 1998 address. But President Bush expressed similar thoughts in 2005 as he sought to generate momentum for change in the Social Security system. Social Security's solvency problem, recognized by both presidents, is not a fundamentally political or partisan issue. Unfortunately, neither president has succeeded in spurring Congress to tackle this pressing problem. Time is slipping away, and it is more urgent than ever to change the course of Social Security in the next few years.

Urging the federal government to initiate changes in its programs is daunting, and implementing these plans will be difficult. Action can be expected when the costs of government programs are forced to the attention of the American body politic.

CHAPTER FIVE

Principles for Reforming Social Security

SOCIAL SECURITY is one of the federal government's most successful programs. It is administered efficiently, and, by and large, it has delivered on its promises. It provides a safety net of retirement income to the nation's elderly and has been so successful in that respect that the poverty rate among the elderly is now lower than among the nonelderly. This wasn't the case before Social Security became large and important in the 1950s and 1960s. Many people now rely on Social Security to provide their basic retirement income.

As we have seen, there is one big problem with Social Security. More promises have been made for the future than the current system has the means to deliver. To put it bluntly, the system is insolvent over the long run—and not by just a little bit. This opinion is not ours alone; it is the opinion of essentially everyone who has closely examined Social Security. The Clinton administration reached this conclusion, as did the subsequent Bush administration. The insolvency of Social Security is not a secret, nor is it controversial. In fact, the annual statements now mailed to every Social Security partici- pant carry this warning in boldface type: **"Your esti- mated benefits are based on current law. Congress has made changes to the law in the past and can do so at any time. The law governing benefit amounts may change because, by 2040, the payroll taxes collected will be enough to pay only about 74 percent of sched- uled benefits."** This official warning is sobering for today's middle-aged and young people who will still be participating in Social Security in 2040, and the trouble is that the solvency problem will surface long before then.

The focus of this chapter and the next is what to do about this serious problem. One thing should be clear at the outset: Doing nothing—more or less the sum of the policy actions of the last twenty years—is not an option. The problem won't go away by ignoring it. A sudden 26 percent across-the-board benefit cut, which is what the boldface warning hints at, would be terrible policy and cause serious problems for both retirees and workers. Remember the famous football coach, George Allen, who, when asked if he was building for the future, said, "The future is now." Well, now is the time to get going on reform of the Social Security system.

We shall first describe how Social Security works. Before evaluating various alternatives for reform, it helps to understand how the system operates now. We'll pay particular attention to whether benefit levels for workers of today and the future can increase as fast as wages or prices. This may sound like a technical distinction, but it makes a critical difference in terms of the solvency of the entire program.

Then we shall lay out some principles for reform. The obvious objective is to fix the system—to overcome the solvency problem so that the system can bring its promises and resources in line with each other. It doesn't make any sense to send out statements that inform participants of their promised benefits and then warn them that the promises can't be kept. In addition to basic solvency, we shall come up with a number of other important principles for reform.

Finally, in the next chapter we shall present specific proposals for reforming the system. Solvency can be achieved. In fact, the problem can be solved in several different ways. We shall present plans that we think are the best and most practical, but we'll also describe several alternative solutions, any one of which would be infinitely better than doing nothing. There really are no excuses for not fixing Social Security. The problem is well understood, and there is wide argument on the menu of choices available to fix it.

The Nuts and Bolts of Social Security Today

The basic structure of Social Security has not changed since at least the 1983 Greenspan reforms. The focus here is on the retirement program within Social Security, although its survivor and disability benefits are also important. The reform proposals subsequently leave these other parts of the program intact.

The Tax Side

The tax side of the Social Security program is simple. As of 2008, Social Security is financed with a 6.2 percent tax on earnings up to $102,000 per year. Both employee and employer pay this 6.2 percent tax, so the total tax on the first $102,000 of earnings is 12.4 percent. For example, if Sharon made $40,000 in wages in 2008, her payment of Social Security taxes would have been 6.2 percent of $40,000, or $2,480. Her employer would have deducted $2,480 from her checks, leaving her with $37,520, net of Social Security taxes.[1] Actually, her employer would have had to forward $4,960 to Social Security—the $2,480 deducted from her paychecks as well as the 6.2 percent employer's tax. Economists believe that workers such as Sharon actually bear the entire burden of the 12.4 percent tax. If it were not for Social Security, she would have made $42,480 (the amount her employment actually costs her employer) instead of $37,520. The accurate way to look at Sharon's situation, therefore, is that she effectively paid $4,960 in Social Security payroll taxes. To put this figure into further perspective, her federal personal income tax bill would almost certainly be less than that. If she were single with no dependents, had no other income, and

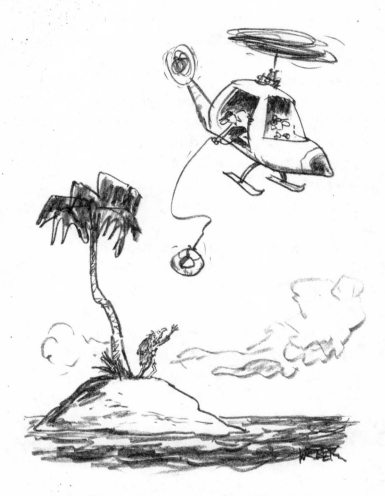

"Forget about me—save Social Security."

relied on the standard deduction, her federal income tax bill would have been $4,451. Like the majority of American workers, she would have paid more in Social Security taxes than in federal income taxes.

These Social Security payroll tax rates have been in effect since 1990 and are not scheduled to change, according to current legislation. However, the maximum level of earnings subject to the full set of taxes, $102,000 for 2008, is raised annually to reflect increases in average wages. The payroll tax has risen dramatically over the years as the program has been scaled up. For instance, the maximum total Social Security tax in 1960 was 6 percent of $4,800, or $288, instead of the 2008 maximum of 12.4 percent of $102,000, or $12,648. The maximum payroll tax payments have gone up forty-four-fold since 1960, while prices have gone up about seven-fold. Any way you look at it, the program has gotten much larger and more expensive.

The Benefit Side

Social Security's retirement benefit structure is much more complicated than the tax structure, and several steps are taken to determine a retiree's initial monthly benefit. First, an individual's record of covered, or taxed, earnings is assembled. Each year of earnings is then multiplied by an average wage index factor. The purpose is to make comparable each year of earnings in an individual's career. For example, if wages in the economy increased by a factor of 6.08 between the year a worker was age twenty-five and the year he was sixty, his earnings at age twenty-five would be multiplied by 6.08 before being compared with his earnings at sixty.

After all wages earned before age sixty are indexed, the next step is to calculate the retiree's average indexed lifetime earnings. This is Social Security's measure of how much a worker earned, on average, in his or her career. First, the highest thirty-five years of indexed earnings—the only years that count—must be identified. If an individual worked for forty-five years, the taxes he or she paid in the ten years with the lowest indexed earnings would not count toward retirement benefits. If the retiree did not work for thirty-five years, some of his or her highest thirty-five years of indexed earnings are simply entered as zeros. Having identified the highest thirty-five years of indexed earnings, Social Security simply adds them up and divides by the number of months in thirty-five years (420). The result is the worker's average indexed monthly earnings, which Social Security refers to as the worker's AIME.[2]

Once the average indexed monthly earnings figure has been computed, we are more than halfway toward figuring out a potential retiree's initial monthly benefit. The next step is to compute the standard monthly benefit amount (termed the primary insurance amount, or PIA), the amount a single retiree would receive per month in initial benefits if he or she retired at the full retirement age. The full retirement age has recently increased to sixty-six for those born from 1943 to 1954. It advances two months per birth year for those born between 1955 and 1960, so for those born in 1960 and later, the full retirement age will be sixty-seven.

The formula that translates the average indexed monthly earnings to the standard monthly benefit amount is progressive; in other words, it offers a more generous conversion for those with low average career earnings than for those with high average earnings. However, when examined on a lifetime basis, the program is less progressive than it appears. The primary reason is that people with low earnings tend to have shorter lives than those with higher incomes. They have a lower chance of collecting any retirement benefits and tend to receive them for shorter intervals once those benefits have commenced.

The final step is to calculate an individual's benefit relative to the benefit if he or she retired at the full retirement age. If an individual retires and claims benefits earlier, his or her monthly benefits will be permanently reduced. On the other hand, for those who begin receiving benefits later than the full retirement age, benefits will be permanently increased, depending on the exact retirement month. The penalty for early retirement and the bonus for late retirement reflect the fact that early retirees will collect benefits longer than

late retirees. Once initial benefits have been determined, future benefits are increased once a year by a
factor determined by price inflation.

There are seemingly endless complications to the full
range of benefit calculations, such as those for widows
and widowers, but you now have the big picture.
Remember one important thing, however: The taxes
described here will not generate enough revenue in the
future to pay the benefits if they are determined in the
manner just explained. Something will have to give, and
it has to be either the benefit determination or the
taxes. Nothing else will bring about solvency.

Wage Indexing Versus Price Indexing

A number of reform or solvency proposals depend on
the way early- and later-career earnings are made comparable. The present system of wage indexing was introduced into the Social Security system in 1977. The
intention was to raise benefits automatically rather than
on an ad hoc basis when politicians got around to it
(almost always in election years). The automatic feature
is a good idea, but tying the increases in initial monthly
benefits to wages has proved unsustainable in the long
run. It is the wage indexing that causes Social Security's
aggregate benefits to grow faster than its tax revenues.
This was foreseen in the report of the officially appointed
Consultant Panel on Social Security, published in August
1976: "The price-indexing method produces expendi-

tures that are relatively level as a percentage of taxable payroll. But the wage-indexing method produces expenditures that require substantially greater tax payments from future generations of workers." The short explanation is that, over time, the Social Security tax base increases with wage growth plus labor force growth, while Social Security retirement benefits under current law increase with wage growth plus beneficiary growth plus growth in life expectancy. The length of retirement has been increasing but the number of years worked has not, so the system's expenditures have grown and will continue to grow faster than revenue.[3] For a business, this would be a ticket to bankruptcy.

In 1976 the Consultant Panel on Social Security correctly predicted that wage indexing would cause insolvency or perpetual shortfalls. Ever since wage indexing was introduced in the United States, twenty-eight out of thirty annual reports by Social Security's trustees have described the system as fiscally insolvent in the long run.

Indexing the automatic increases to price levels rather than wage levels may sound like a small change, but it could have large consequences, as we will discuss in chapter 6. The underlying insight is that, in general, wages go up faster than prices because of productivity increases. If prices were used rather than wages, the rate of increase in future initial monthly benefits would be lower. Still, the price indexing method would preserve the real value of benefits.

Table 5.1 shows the initial monthly benefits for three

Table 5.1 Primary Insurance Amounts If Price Indexing Had Been Adopted in 1983

	CURRENT SYSTEM OF WAGE INDEXING	SYSTEM OF PRICE INDEXING
Individual earns half of national average wage for thirty-five years	$888	$727
Individual earns national average wage for thirty-five years	$1,383	$1,163
Individual earns more than payroll tax cutoff for thirty-five years	$2,120	$1,716

hypothetical individuals who reached the age of sixty-two in 2007. The middle column shows benefits under the current law. The progressivity of the benefit formula is illustrated in that the monthly benefits for someone whose earnings were always at the national average are only 56 percent higher (rather than twice as high) as the benefits for someone who always earned half as much. The right-hand column shows what the benefits would be today if the Social Security Administration had adopted price indexing reform at the time of the Greenspan Commission in 1983. The numbers in this column could be called "what if" numbers. The table shows that benefits would be 16 to 19 percent lower for someone reaching the age of sixty-two in 2007 if the government had switched to price indexing in 1984. Current retirees might consider themselves lucky, but if that switch had been made, Social Security would be completely solvent today rather than being several trillion dollars short.

Western Europe, where an aging population and other demographic developments create more immediate pressures than in the United States, has largely been forced to abandon wage indexing. The United Kingdom took significant action earlier than most countries and, in 1980, switched from wage indexing to price indexing for its basic state pension.[4] In 1992 and 1993, Italy and France, respectively, passed legislation to switch from wage indexing to price indexing.[5] Germany introduced a "sustainability factor" in the benefit calculations for its state pensions in 2004.[6] Essentially, the German government will pay benefits only out of the money that is available, and there will be less available than would be needed to pay wage-indexed benefits.

With this background on how the current system works and the need for change to achieve solvency, we propose five general principles for any economically and politically acceptable reform proposal.

1. Those individuals nearing retirement age should be guaranteed benefits as provided under current law.

This guarantee is widely agreed upon. It would apply to all who are fifty-five years of age or older because they have too little time to make alternative plans. As many in this age group count on Social Security, any change in the rules should be gradual and announced far in advance. Every serious proposal should protect those over fifty-five from changes in benefits.

2. **Low-income individuals should be protected, and the progressivity of Social Security should be maintained or even enhanced.**

For 65 percent of beneficiaries, Social Security benefit payments provide more than half their total retirement income. For 21 percent of beneficiaries, Social Security is the only source of income. The safety net that Social Security provides in old age is substantial, and reform proposals should maintain and strengthen this safety net. Those who experience low lifetime earnings should not be made worse off than they are under the current law.

3. **The rate of growth of benefits must be contained.**

This issue is more complex but just as compelling as the two previous points. The Social Security program's projected finances are such that the income it receives is a constant percentage of total payroll. However, benefits are projected to be an increasingly larger percentage of total payroll. Chart 5.1 illustrates this point. It shows the income and costs of Social Security as a percentage of the total covered payroll. The income rate consists mostly of the total payroll taxes received from employees and employers. The cost rate is the amount paid out to beneficiaries as a percentage of covered payroll. The shortfall of income relative to costs over the next seventy-five years gives a sense of the financial troubles of these programs. In 2006 this shortfall of Social Security was estimated to be 2.02 percent of taxable payroll over the next seventy-five years.[7]

Chart 5.1 Cost and Income Rates of Social Security

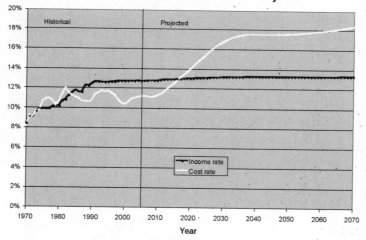

It is clear that the Greenspan Commission accomplished something important in 1983. Before that, from the mid-1970s to 1983, Social Security was running substantial deficits. In fact, by 1983 Social Security was on the verge of having to delay or reduce benefits. The system almost ran out of money. Then, with the reforms of Social Security in 1983, the system swung into surplus and has been in that situation ever since. But the surplus will begin to shrink dramatically in just a couple of years and will disappear completely by 2017. After that, the projections are for deficits as far as the eye can see. But, it is even worse than that: Not only is the cost rate higher than the income rate beginning in 2017, but the cost rate is increasing much more rapidly than the income rate. This means that tax increases alone will not solve the financial problems of Social Security. Increasing taxes is merely a temporary fix for a permanent problem. If tax rates in 2070 were increased to the projected cost rate of a little over 18 percent, with no other changes to benefits, the system would immediately step out of balance in 2071 because the benefits paid are projected to increase faster than the tax base. The only way to solve the problem is to adjust the growth rate of costs by introducing changes that prevent the programs' costs from growing more quickly than their tax bases (aggregate covered earnings).

4. Individual retirement accounts should be considered.
Individual accounts have considerable merit as part of Social Security reform. They cannot cure the solvency problem—in fact, they are almost always solvency neutral, neither worsening nor helping with that issue—but they certainly can help increase the saving rate in a country that needs more saving. They would encourage or even require citizens to participate in American capitalism. This is sometimes called the

ownership advantage. And the return on private U.S. markets has historically been very attractive.

Many alternatives exist for the size and structure of private accounts. They could be funded in whole or in part from a portion of the payroll taxes paid on behalf of an individual, with defined benefits reduced commensurably, a practice known as a carve-out. The alternative would be an addition to the payroll tax, called an add-on, as the source of funds. Our own view is that individual accounts, if adopted, should be substantial in size in order to justify the extra costs of setting up and administering the system. No doubt, investment choices would be limited to well-diversified options in order to control risk, and the allocation between equity and fixed income funds would change as an individual ages.

One advantage of individual accounts is that contributions to them are far less distorting than are payroll taxes. Even mandatory contributions to an individual account should not be considered as taxes. The money still belongs to the owner of the account, who typically has some control over how funds are invested and can either enjoy the proceeds in retirement or bequeath them to heirs. Another advantage of individual accounts is that they contain real assets, such as stocks and bonds. In addition, once the funds are identified as being owned by an individual, the likelihood that those funds could be spent as though they were general revenue, as are the current trust funds, would be minimal.

5. Social Security should be flexible to adjust to future demographic and economic shifts.

Many of Social Security's financial problems stem from a fundamentally positive fact: Life expectancies have increased dramatically, as shown in chapter 1, and are projected to continue to increase in the future. Nevertheless, mortality rates, fertility rates, and other demographic characteristics are difficult to predict with any amount of accuracy. In 1977, when wage indexing was introduced as a way to increase benefits automatically to maintain the standard of living of beneficiaries, the rate of price growth was higher than wage growth. Today that relationship has reversed. The Social Security system can adapt to many of these changes only with new legislation, so policy makers must regard the system as a work in progress and be ready to take action at appropriate times. Senators Dianne Feinstein and Pete Domenici introduced legislation along these lines in January 2007. They would have a commission appointed with the mandate to review the system continuously and recommend appropriate changes periodically. The legislation encourages Congress to move expeditiously on entitlement reform.

The following chapter presents reform plans that meet the general principles outlined above and promise to eliminate the long-run solvency problem. There is a menu of several possible solutions that would work. The challenge is to find the best set of adjustments to transform the present unsustainable program into a system that is sound and solvent.

CHAPTER SIX

Plans for Reforming Social Security

SOCIAL SECURITY as it stands is insolvent. As we have seen, the program's administrators say as much in each of the more than one hundred million statements they send out each year to participants. Fixing Social Security's solvency is a major task, but it can be done, and it should be done promptly. It is only fair to American workers that they should know how this problem is going to be solved in order to plan their careers, their retirements, and their saving strategies.

Social Security can be made solvent without raising taxes, and that is the strategy we advocate. This implies that our proposals focus on the benefit side. There are several reasons why we favor this approach. First, the system promises higher real benefits for future retirees than it pays today's retirees. Therefore, benefit increases could be cut while maintaining their current level. Second, higher taxes create a drag on the economy, so we view raising taxes as a last resort. Third, we need to keep our powder dry in terms of increasing tax rates because the government health insurance programs, Medicare and Medicaid, which will be discussed in Part III, are likely to have escalating costs even after their benefit structure is improved. As much as possible, we should not resort to tax increases to solve our problems because doing so will create an even bigger potential problem: a slow-growing, even stagnant, economy.

If we assume that we choose to live within the means of the current 12.4 percent payroll tax, the variables that can be combined in any option to achieve solvency are these: (1) The indexing system could be changed so that the rate of increase in benefit levels over and above inflation is either eliminated or moderated; (2) the age at which full benefit payments commence could be raised; and (3) some form of individual accounts could be introduced with the possibility of an additional payroll deduction on a mandatory or voluntary basis.

We begin by putting on the table two options that retain the defined benefit nature of Social Security, protect the poor, increase the progressivity of the system, and are introduced gradually.[1] They meet the goal of solvency and score well against the principles that we presented in the last chapter. The first option, called Progressive Price Indexing Plus, stays within the framework of the present system. The second plan involves large, mandatory individual accounts. We call this option the Personal Security Account plan.[2] Although the level of defined benefits now promised by the federal government would be restructured, the overall retirement resources delivered by Social Security, including the associated individual accounts, would likely be at least as large as those currently promised.

These are by no means the only options. We shall also identify, as points of departure for debate, other reform proposals that combine several of the features of Progressive Price Indexing Plus and Personal Security Accounts and offer alternative paths to Social Security solvency.

Progressive Price Indexing Plus

As described in chapter 5, initial Social Security old-age benefits increase with the average level of wages in the economy, and wages tend to rise faster than prices over the long run because the economy enjoys productivity improvements. Some of these improvements are due to more and better tools for workers, such as computers and associated software, and others are due to widespread advances in education. The net result of wage indexing initial benefits is that future beneficiaries—our children and grandchildren—are being promised higher monthly benefits in inflation-adjusted terms than today's Social Security beneficiaries receive. Because the rate of increase of the system's promised benefits must be moderated to restore its solvency, a good way to start is by trimming the rate of increase in future real benefits that the system now promises. As with a private pension plan under financial pressure, Social Security should not propose an increase in future benefits when it faces insolvency.

Progressive price indexing changes the way future benefits are calculated in different ways for different individuals. It would leave the benefit calculation, described in chapter 5, unchanged for everyone in the bottom 30 percent of the lifetime earnings distribution. That is, the lowest 30 percent of the population in terms of lifetime labor income would continue to have the level of its initial benefits grow with the average wage rate in the economy. That meets one of our principles of not reducing the benefits of those with relatively low incomes. However, workers with the highest lifetime incomes (those whose earnings were at or above the Social Security earnings cap for most of their career) would have their benefits grow only as fast as prices. Those beneficiaries between the lowest 30 percent of earners and these top-earning individuals would see their benefits rise faster than prices but slower than wages. Another important fact is that none of today's retirees would ever have their benefits reduced from the level that is currently promised, and the plan would be introduced gradually.

Let's take the case in which wages triple by 2050 while prices double. If that happens between now and then, the Federal Reserve will have done a very good job in controlling inflation, and real wages would have increased by 50 percent. Under progressive price index-ing, the Social Security benefits of those in the bottom 30 percent of lifetime earnings would triple. Their real benefits would be 50 percent higher than today's retirees who were in a similar position in the distribu-tion of average indexed lifetime earnings. Those at the top of the earnings distribution would have double the benefits of today's retirees, just matching inflation. Those in between would enjoy benefits somewhere between two and three times as high as today's Social Security recipients. We think of this blend as progres-sive price indexing.

This approach further increases the progressivity of the system because those who receive low monthly ben-efits would have more rapidly growing benefits than those receiving high monthly benefits. Eventually, in ninety or one hundred years or perhaps longer, the benefit level would be the same for most Social Security participants, and it would be at the real level of the highest benefit received today. Productivity would per-mit almost everyone three or four generations from now to receive the maximum benefits paid out today even after adjustment for inflation.

Now we get to the "plus" part of the plan. Progressive price indexing alone goes only about three-quarters of the way toward completely restoring the solvency of Social Security. How can solvency be achieved without raising tax rates? It should not come as any surprise to those who have read this far that we favor closing the rest of the gap by increasing the age at which Social Security beneficiaries can claim full benefits.

Right now, the full-benefit retirement age is scheduled to advance to sixty-seven by 2023 and remain at that age forever. While it may appear that nothing is forever, the full retirement age stayed at sixty-five from 1935 until 2000. We don't think that it should get stuck again, this time at sixty-seven, so we suggest that after 2023, the full retirement age advance by the amount of the increase in life expectancy of sixty-seven-year-olds. That is, if by 2040 the life expectancy of sixty-seven-year-olds has increased by one year relative to where it was in 2023, the full retirement age would be increased by one year to sixty-eight. In all probability, the age at which full benefits could be claimed would increase by a month every year or two. All the adjustments would be very gradual, and the average length of retirement would not be reduced. Combining changes in retirement age and changes in wage and price indexing accomplishes the goal of restoring the system's solvency.

We now have all the pieces of the Progressive Price Indexing Plus plan in place: a strong shift from wage to price indexing across most income categories, retention of wage indexing—and hence progressivity—at the lowest income levels, plus a gradual increase in the age of retirement. It does the job in terms of solvency, but it does not dramatically change the structure of Social Security. For instance, it would not necessarily improve saving incentives in a country that clearly needs to increase saving. It modifies the existing system but retains the defined benefit, or defined promise, system that is rapidly becoming obsolete in the private sector.

This is where individual accounts come in. Adding them would be straightforward. They could be, as described in chapter 5, add-on or carve-out accounts as long as they do not worsen the solvency of the whole package. They could be created on a voluntary or mandatory basis. Supplemental accounts, in particular, would allow those whose promised benefits do not rise at the presently scheduled rate to make up the difference in their retirement resources. It is our view that adding individual accounts to this proposed system would be economically and politically attractive once the basic solvency of the system was assured.

Personal Security Account

A quite different approach to Social Security solvency is known as the Personal Security Account plan. We consider this plan to be as appealing as the Progressive Price Indexing Plus plan, but it is a more radical reform and might be less viable politically. It protects and strengthens the redistribution inherent in the Social Security system and the safety net that it offers those with low lifetime labor earnings. It would also enhance the saving rate in the United States. The plan is actually composed of two pieces: an extremely progressive defined benefit system and large, mandatory defined contribution individual accounts. As with Progressive Price Indexing Plus, this plan would be introduced very gradually as the old system was phased out.

The basic structure of the Personal Security Account plan is quite simple and consists of two parts:

1. A completely flat benefit amount for those with full careers. That is, CEOs and janitors would receive exactly the same flat monthly benefit. The amount would be $600 per month per participant in 2007, an amount that would be wage-indexed in the future. Two-earner couples, in which both spouses worked full-length careers, would receive $1,200 per month.

2. A mandatory Personal Security Account with annual contributions equal to 5 percent of salary. This would be funded with a required additional contribution of 2.5 percent of salary from workers and 2.5 percent of salary from existing payroll tax receipts.

Certainly, $600 per month is a modest sum. However, let's put the generosity of this plan in perspective. The average benefit today is approximately $1,000 per month. The Personal Security Account plan with its $600-per-month flat benefit and its 5 percent individual accounts would almost surely result in higher average monthly benefits than those provided under current-law Social Security.

Participants would have choices for investing in their 5 percent accounts ranging from safe, long-term, inflation-protected Treasury securities to broadly diversified, or indexed, equity funds. We would favor a menu of choices approved by the government, which would require all offerings to have relatively low fees. Expenses could be capped at 1 percent per year, and competition would undoubtedly encourage many funds to offer even lower fees.

The Personal Security Accounts would be used exclusively for retirement savings and could not be used for other purposes, such as home purchases, medical expenses, or collateral for loans. In that sense, they would be similar to current Social Security benefits. Such restrictions would ensure that the funds in these accounts would be available for retirement savings. Any balances remaining at death could be bequeathed to heirs. As in the Progressive Price Indexing Plus plan, this plan would index the retirement age with life expectancy starting in 2023.

If we assume that wages grow an average 1 percent per year faster than prices, the $600 per month offered as the first tier of the Personal Security Account plan would increase to almost $1,000 per month by 2050. Under the Personal Security Account plan, total benefits for low- and moderate-income participants would be higher than benefits under the current Social Security system updated to 2050, even when we assume a very conservative return of 2.2 percent over inflation on individual accounts. With a still-conservative 4 percent real return, which might be earned after expenses on a fifty-fifty stock-bond portfolio, everyone would enjoy total benefits exceeding those currently promised.

While it is very likely that the Personal Security Account plan would result in greater retirement wealth for individuals, more savings for the economy, and a Social Security system that is solvent in the long run, these accomplishments should not be thought of as remarkable or free. In order to achieve these positive results, workers would not only pay current Social Security payroll taxes but also make a mandatory 2.5 percent contribution to their individual accounts on the first $102,000 of earnings, a figure that would be increased each year as average wages rise, just as under current law.

Nothing is free in terms of restoring Social Security's solvency, and the Personal Security Account plan cannot get around that fact. Any plan that does not reduce the expected future benefit promises of the current system would have to identify additional sources of revenue at least as great as the new 2.5 percent mandatory contributions of the Personal Security Account plan.

Progressive Price Indexing Plus Versus Personal Security Accounts

The Progressive Price Indexing Plus plan reduces the rate of increase in benefits while holding the payroll tax rates financing Social Security at a fixed level. The Personal Security Account plan requires larger contributions from workers. There is no magic in the way it maintains and potentially enhances benefits, in part by increasing the funding of the system and in part by sensibly investing the additional funds. The Personal Security Account plan would transfer a significant part of Social Security payments to a Personal Security Account system in which the amount of benefits would directly reflect the amount of contributions. This plan would likely increase national saving, which in turn would increase national income in the future.

These two plans represent two different types of available sensible choices. One gradually reduces the rate of increase in benefits promised to those above the bottom 30 percent of the lifetime earnings distribution to fit within the parameters of projected payroll tax receipts; the other offers the prospect of benefits at least as high as current promises but requires additional contributions from workers. The Personal Security Account system could be added to the structure of the Progressive Price Indexing Plus plan. Selecting either approach in the next few years would be vastly better than doing nothing for another decade or longer and then facing the music. Of course there are many other possibilities.

Other Alternatives for Social Security Reform

President George W. Bush appointed a Commission on Social Security that set out several proposals in 2001.[3] The commission's so-called Reform Model 2 would achieve solvency primarily by replacing wage indexing with price indexing for everyone under the age of fifty-five. Consider once again the scenario in which wages triple by 2050, whereas prices double from today's level. The current law, which uses wage indexing, promises to triple Social Security benefits, whereas the commission's Reform Model 2 would double the monetary payments by using price indexing. Chapter 5 showed how powerful such a switch in indexing methods could be; the difference between the two would completely restore solvency. In fact, solvency would be more than restored, and thus Reform Model 2 was able to propose a new minimum for those who work full-time at the minimum wage for at least thirty years. Benefits for individuals who fall in this category would be increased to at least 120 percent of the poverty level. Individual accounts would be an option for workers under fifty-five years of age, who would be allowed to redirect to personal accounts 4 percent of their payroll taxes, up to an annual maximum of $1,000. If an individual chose to redirect money into his individual account, his defined benefit payments would be lowered accordingly. The commission estimates that this approach "enables all future retirees to receive an inflation-adjusted Social Security benefit that is at least as great as today's retirees."[4]

Our view is that Reform Model 2 of the president's commission has a lot of merit. It restores solvency, protects those over fifty-five, improves the treatment of those with the lowest lifetime earnings, and introduces voluntary individual accounts. Its quick adoption would have been a big improvement from the do-nothing path we seem to be on. However, we believe that capping the contributions to individual accounts at $1,000 is a mistake. Individual accounts are like many things in life. If you are going to use them, you should do so on a reasonable scale. So our approach would add to that plan significant individual accounts, as set out earlier in our Personal Security Account plan.

Congressman Rahm Emanuel, now chairman of the House Democratic Caucus, has recently proposed an interesting version of personal accounts in a *Wall Street Journal* article entitled "Supplementing Social Security." In his words,

> Building on the principles of personal accounts, universal savings and the desire in the marketplace for simplicity, I believe we should create Universal Savings Accounts. Like 401(k)s, the accounts would supplement Social Security. Employers and employees would contribute 1 percent of paychecks on a tax-deductible basis. Additional contributions could be made to the accounts at the discretion of the company or individual worker.

To ensure low management fees, these accounts would be managed by the private sector but overseen by a quasi-public board that would be given fiduciary responsibility for the types of investment options that workers could select. . . .

To help achieve universal participation and simplicity, employers would automatically enroll their employees in these accounts, allowing employees to opt out if they decided that they did not want to participate. Amounts contributed could be automatically increased and account balances invested in "lifecycle funds," ensuring that individuals are making appropriate investment decisions based on their age.[5]

A different alternative for Social Security reform has been presented by Martin Feldstein and Andrew Samwick, longtime scholars of the Social Security system.[6] Under the Feldstein-Samwick proposal, the growth rate of pay-as-you-go benefits would be slowed gradually "up to a cumulative maximum reduction of 40 percent from the benchmark level of benefits." They estimate that this 40 percent gap would be more than filled by the combination of a 1.5 percent transfer from the payroll tax and an additional matching 1.5 percent that individuals would contribute on a voluntary out-of-pocket basis. According to Feldstein and Samwick, "A portfolio invested 60 percent in the Standard and Poor's 500 index of common stocks and 40 percent in a portfolio of corporate bonds during the 50-year period through 1995 had a mean real return of 6.9 percent." They use this return in calculating the values generated in their proposed personal accounts. The result would have personal accounts more than make up for the reduction in traditional Social Security benefits. Note that if we had used the assumed rate of return of 6.9 percent in the Personal Security Account plan, the benefit levels would have been raised significantly. Feldstein and Samwick also examine such issues as administrative costs, risks, and income distribution effects. When evaluating their proposal, it is important to remember, as with all others, that the status quo—standing pat with the current law—is not an option.

Another plan that shares many elements with those already discussed is Peter G. Peterson's proposal in his book *Running on Empty*. Peterson, a longtime and persistent crusader for attention to the coming costs of our Social Security and health care systems, favors a switch to price indexing similar to the proposal in Reform Model 2 of the president's commission, but he includes mandatory, rather than voluntary, add-on personal accounts. Under his plan the government would provide an improved safety net for low-income workers by contributing to their personal accounts.

One final plan that deserves mention was proposed by the scholars Peter Diamond and Peter Orszag in *Saving Social Security: A Balanced Approach*. Their plan restores long-run solvency to Social Security through a combination of tax increases and benefit reductions. First, they suggest that an automatic adjustment be built into Social

Security for advances in life expectancy. Each year, Social Security would calculate the extra costs associated with lower mortality rates over the past year. Half of this cost would be borne by workers aged fifty-nine and younger in the form of reduced benefits, and the other half would be offset by an increased payroll tax rate. Second, Diamond and Orszag favor increasing the maximum taxable earnings base gradually over time. Third, they would increase the progressivity of the system by slightly reducing benefits for high earners. Fourth, they would increase payroll taxes and reduce benefits by roughly 0.30 percent each year beginning in 2023 and introduce a new "legacy tax" on earnings above the maximum taxable earnings base of approximately 3 percent.

Our view is that the Diamond-Orszag proposal relies too heavily on tax increases. But at least it grapples with the solvency issue and comes up with a package of changes that would make the system financially stable.

Many other routes to Social Security reform are possible. The features of the reform plans that we have described can be combined as long as the goal of achieving solvency is kept in mind. For instance, large voluntary individual accounts could be added to the Progressive Indexing Plus plan, combining some of the features of the Personal Security Account plan, the Progressive Price Indexing Plus plan, and the Reform Model 2 plan of the president's commission.

The lesson from this mix-and-match exercise is that a set of ingredients is already available that can be combined to restore Social Security's solvency and make the system work more effectively for the economy and for its participants. We should demand action on Social Security; the problem is well understood and the choices are well defined. A new and solvent system could be hammered out in a matter of months if we, as a country, put our minds to it.

Solvent Alternatives

Progressive Price Indexing Plus	Keep wage indexing for lowest 30 percent, phase in price indexing for those at higher levels, and index age of full benefits to longevity changes. Can be combined with matched 2.5 percentage points of payroll tax to personal accounts.
Personal Security Account	Combine low flat benefit that is wage indexed with matched 2.5 percentage points of payroll tax to personal accounts, and index age of full benefits to longevity changes.
President's Commission on Social Security: Reform Model 2	Switch to price indexing with unused money devoted to new minimum for low-income workers. Option to redirect up to 4 percentage points of payroll tax to personal accounts up to a maximum of $1,000 per year.
Rahm Emanuel	Introduce Universal Savings Accounts financed by matched 1 percentage point of payroll tax and invested in "life cycle funds."
Feldstein & Samwick	Reduce current benefit levels gradually by 40 percent, and invest a matched 1.5 percentage points of a payroll tax to private accounts to make up for shortfall.
Peter G. Peterson	Switch to price indexing with add-on creation of personal accounts with safety net for low-income workers.
Diamond & Orszag	Achieve long-run solvency through a combination of benefit reductions and tax increases.

PART THREE

America's System
of Health Care

CHAPTER SEVEN

The Past Is Prologue

HEALTH IS A UNIQUE and personal subject. People everywhere, and certainly Americans, respond almost instinctively to health needs. A natural or man-made catastrophe somehow always seems to bring out the best in our human nature, and we reach out to those in need. We expect medical services to be broadly available and of high quality.

But a tipping point is now at hand. The costs of the U.S. health care system are wildly high by international standards and are rising rapidly. At more than 16 percent of the GDP, the cost of U.S. health care exceeds that of any other developed country by one-third and is, for instance, roughly double the percentage spent in Great Britain.[1] Costs have escalated so rapidly in recent years that by 2006 they had doubled as a percentage of GDP from their 1975 level. This trend is not confined to the United States. In fact, health care costs as a percentage of GDP are rising steadily in all developed countries.

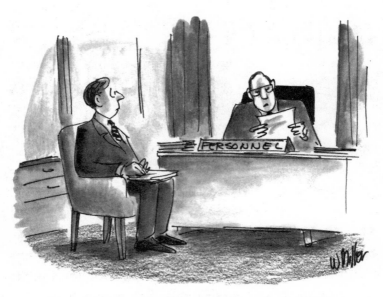

*"Of course, with the position that has the benefits—
medical, dental, et cetera—there is no salary."*

Looked at another way, health insurance premiums in most years since 1988 have increased at rates double or triple those of general inflation or earnings.[2] This means that each year health insurance premiums are taking up a greater percentage of an individual's income (whether paid directly by the employee or indirectly through the employer), leaving a smaller share for all other expenditures. Certainly, one reason that all too many people lack health insurance coverage is that they are simply priced out of the market.

Health insurance costs cannot continue to grow faster than wages forever.

The increase in health care spending has two possible explanations, one benign and the other worrisome. The benign explanation is that as a society grows richer and older and develops new technology, individuals choose to spend more money on health care, including such things as new antibiotics, vaccines, and pacemakers. If this benign explanation is accurate, then rising spending on health care might not be a problem at all. But the worrisome explanation is that health care spending is rising because of an inefficient system that wastes money and forces us to spend more on health care than we really wish to spend. If the second explanation is correct and there are no brakes on rising health care spending, then eventually a financial crisis will ensue as other important economic expenditure categories are crowded out.

The source of rising health care costs undoubtedly involves both explanations. A significant body of evidence suggests that while much new health care spending is worthwhile, a substantial amount of it is wasted. A research study on regional variations in Medicare payments suggests that approximately 30 percent of Medicare expenditures lead to no improvements in health.[3] Projections of Medicare costs reveal a system that is out of control and not even close to living within its means. Likewise, health insurance premiums rise dramatically year after year, and 40 percent of Americans are dissatisfied with their own health care costs.[4]

In light of these facts, can the quality and accessibility of the U.S. health care system be preserved and enhanced while escalating costs are brought under control? The answer must be yes because cost projections show that health care expenditures will take over this country's large and rising gross domestic product unless changes are made.

A vast body of literature exists on the development of health care in America.[5] This chapter, drawing on that literature, traces the historical pattern leading to current developments, presents a picture of where matters stand today, and identifies areas of large and unnecessary costs. Chapter 8 calls attention to the dramatic impact of domestic and international research and development on health. Chapter 9 examines areas where cost pressures are producing changes in the health care system and considers the questions raised most insistently about the effectiveness of that system.

Then chapter 10 evaluates emerging alternatives to the present health care system to determine which of them deserve support and further action. Chosen with care, one or more of these alternatives would lead to an improved system that can provide high-quality health care and bring costs under control.

Some History

The history of health insurance has its beginnings in the 1920s. It evolved during the 1930s as insurance plans were established to cover hospital costs, and it grew during the Great Depression. Eventually various plans were combined under the auspices of the American Hospital Association (AHA) and became known as Blue Cross. These Blue Cross plans, considered socially desirable because they provided benefits to people in need, benefited from special state-sponsored legislation that made them tax-exempt, nonprofit corporations. As such, they were freed from insurance regulations demanding high reserves, but they were burdened by their obligation to sell health insurance to anyone who wished to purchase a policy. High-risk individuals were more likely to purchase insurance coverage because they saw the plan as a good deal. This tendency, known as adverse selection, had the effect of forcing Blue Cross to set a high price for insurance coverage.[6]

Commercial insurance companies had long been reluctant to enter the health care market. They did so, however, when they realized how to avoid adverse selection: They offered insurance through employers to groups of working individuals, most of whom were relatively young and healthy.

The health insurance system took off during World War II, when wages and prices were controlled but benefits were not. To compete for employees in a tight labor market, employers looked elsewhere and realized they could offer to provide health insurance, among other inducements, as a substitute for banned wage increases. By this time, commercial insurers were ready to go. These alternative forms of compensation were not regarded as taxable income, so employers bought insurance policies and their employees could access the health care system using pretax dollars without incurring significant out-of-pocket expenses.[7] As the system evolved and as the tax advantage of employment-based health insurance stimulated its use, the dominant players came to be the employers (those who provided the money) and the insurers and medical professionals (those who provided the services). Beneficiaries of the health care system, the patients, had little incentive to evaluate relative costs or to take the outlook of a normal consumer, while they had every incentive to use the system without restraint because they did not directly bear a significant fraction of the costs.

With the jump start provided by the World War II wage and price controls, the support of labor unions, and the tax-advantaged status of benefits, employment-based health coverage grew by leaps and bounds in the second half of the twentieth century. By 2003, employment-based health insurance covered approximately 160 million people, or nearly three of every five nonelderly Americans.[8]

Beginning in 1965, the federal government emerged as a major financier of medical services. Established by legislation that President Johnson signed with a flourish in 1965, Medicare is a health program for individuals over the age of sixty-five, and Medicaid is a joint federal-state health program targeted toward the poor and disabled. Initially, both programs followed the general pattern of employment-based insurance in the sense that an eligible person was entitled to receive a set of covered medical services while paying only modest fees.

Medicaid

By 2004, Medicaid spending had risen to $287 billion, with $115 billion spent by the states and $172 billion by the federal government.[9] Just two years later, in 2006, the total had grown to approximately $350 billion. More than one in every six Americans is a recipient of Medicaid.

Nonetheless, not all individuals who qualify for Medicaid are enrolled in the program. In fact, some studies estimate that approximately 20 percent of uninsured children are eligible for Medicaid but not enrolled.[10] It is not surprising that uninsured adults who are eligible for, but not enrolled in, Medicaid have fewer health problems than adults who are enrolled in the program.[11] Many individuals and families do not realize they are eligible for Medicaid or wait to sign up until they encounter health problems.

Medicaid is actually composed of fifty-six separate entities because each state and territory administers its own unique program.[12] In order to qualify for federal support, a state's Medicaid program must cover a number of services such as inpatient and outpatient hospital treatment, prenatal care, children's vaccines, and nursing homes. The state then receives federal matching funds for all the Medicaid services it delivers. States also receive federal matching funds if they provide a variety of optional services such as diagnostic tests, prosthetic devices, and optometry services. States must apply for waivers if they wish to depart, even slightly, from the basic structure of Medicaid.

Medicaid does not provide money to Medicaid beneficiaries but pays doctors and health care providers directly for services rendered. Copayments or other cost-sharing arrangements are limited by law to extremely low levels.

Eligibility requirements for Medicaid differ by state, but in general they are based on income level, value of personal assets, age, and whether an individual is blind, disabled, or pregnant. Children make up the largest group of Medicaid enrollees (48 percent) whereas the disabled receive the largest component of spending (43 percent). A significant portion of Medicaid funds (28 percent) goes to the aged, including dual-eligible individuals—those low-income elderly who are eligible for both Medicare and Medicaid. Medicaid also plays a large role in such specific health care areas as prenatal and long-term care, and it provides financial support for more than one-third of all births in the United States.[13]

Flush with cash during boom times in the late 1990s, many states expanded their Medicaid programs by reducing eligibility requirements and increasing coverage for optional services. Since then, health costs have continued to rise while increases in tax revenue to states have declined from the giddy days of the late 1990s. One unnerving result is that 2003 was the first year in which states, taken as a whole, spent more on Medicaid than they did on K–12 education. Medicaid spending growth has slowed recently from 12 percent per annum in 2000–2002 to 8.1 percent per annum in 2003–2004, but these rates of increase are still well in excess of the rates of inflation or the growth in wages.[14]

In 2004, Medicaid paid for 42 percent of the $158 billion spent on long-term care while Medicare paid for another 20 percent.[15] Nursing home care, the single largest component of long-term care, totaled $115 billion in 2004.[16]

In one of many efforts to control spending growth, states and the federal government have been tightening rules to combat various Medicaid-planning strategies by which patients in need of long-term care transfer their assets to family members in order to qualify for Medicaid. The federal government's Deficit Reduction Act (DRA) of 2005 lengthened various income lookback periods and tightened eligibility rules to combat this type of abuse. It is not yet clear if the DRA will substantially alleviate the problem or if, over time, people will again outfox the system.

Medicare

Medicare, a federal health care program for individuals aged sixty-five and over, is composed of four parts, known by the first four letters of the alphabet. Part A provides hospital insurance and is financed by a 2.9 percent payroll tax. Part B covers doctor visits and a variety of outpatient treatments and is financed by premiums paid by the individual and general government revenues. Part C, otherwise known as Medicare Advantage, allows seniors to receive government Medicare in the structure of a health maintenance organization (HMO) and is financed by a combination of premiums, 2.9 percent of payroll tax, and general government revenues. Part D provides a prescription drug benefit and is also financed by premiums and general government revenues.

Individuals aged sixty-five years or older become eligible if they or their spouses worked in Medicare-covered employment for at least ten years. Kidney dialysis patients or those who have received Social Security disability payments for at least two years are also eligible.

As of 2006, 43 million people, including seniors and the disabled, were enrolled in Part A (hospital insurance); 40 million in Part B (doctor visits and outpatient treatments); 6.6 million in Part C (the alternative HMO structure); and 28 million in Part D (the new prescription drug benefit).[17]

The federal government spent $408 billion, or 3.1 percent of GDP, on Medicare in 2006, and the Con-

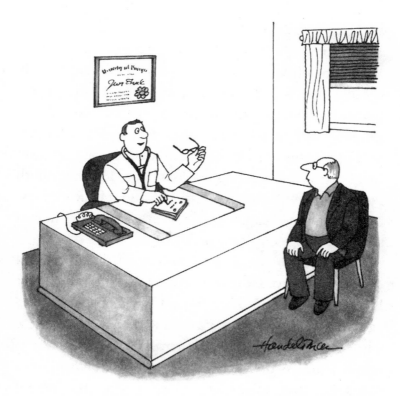

"*You're in luck, in a way. Now is the time to be sick—while Medicare still has some money.*"

gressional Budget Office (CBO) projects that this figure will reach 4 percent by 2015. Medicare receives more federal funds than Medicaid does, but in terms of combined state and federal spending, Medicaid is larger than Medicare.

Another important feature of Medicare's cost structure is that, like Medicaid, a relatively small number of cases account for a large proportion of Medicare's costs. The costliest 5 percent of Medicare recipients account for 43 percent of Medicare's costs and have average yearly spending of $63,000 a person. The least expensive 50 percent account for 3.8 percent of Medicare's costs and have average yearly spending of $550 a person. Medicaid, not Medicare, is the primary source of funding for long-term care because the low-income elderly can qualify for both programs simultaneously and because Medicare contributes only to relatively short stays in nursing homes and other long-term care facilities.

Over time, Medicare's premiums, deductibles, and copayments have become more significant, at least for high-income elderly Americans. Part A, hospital coverage, is available without a monthly premium for those who have paid the Medicare payroll tax for a minimum of ten years. As of 2008, the Part A deductible amount was $1,024 per hospital stay, meaning that the patient pays the first $1,024 of the total bill. For the first sixty days of a hospital stay, Medicare pays all covered costs above the deductible without copayments.

Part B, which is often called medical insurance in contrast to hospital insurance covered by Part A, had a basic monthly premium of $96.40 per month as of 2008. This premium is higher for single people with incomes in excess of $80,000 and for married couples with incomes in excess of $160,000. For those high-income elderly, the monthly premium is gradually escalated as income goes up until the premium reaches $238.40 per month. Part B also features an annual $135 deductible and a 20 percent copayment for all Medicare-covered services. Part D, the relatively new prescription drug program, offers a wide variety of plans, but most involve monthly premiums, deductible amounts, and copayment charges.

Because of these deductibles and copayments in Parts A, B, and D, as well as some perceived gaps in coverage, many elderly individuals buy supplemental private so-called Medigap policies. The copayment features of Parts B and D have the advantage of encouraging people to be more thoughtful about their use of medical care inasmuch as they must make some contribution to the cost of the drugs or services. However, all reformers of entitlement programs need to keep in mind the welfare of the low-income elderly and the potential burden of the copayments and deductibles. This is one of the reasons that several of the Social Security reform proposals discussed in the last chapter protected the lifetime poor from benefit cuts and thereby increased the progressivity of the system.

Indicators of Large Unnecessary Costs

Any system that allows, and even encourages, people to use its services at a small fraction of cost to them will produce a few predictable results:

1. Liberal legitimate use of services the system was created to provide, a use that forms the basis of strong political support for its continuation.

2. Concern among payers about costs, leading to numerous and varied controls, particularly on prices of services provided, and the emergence of unproductive competition among providers of services and providers of money over who will pay and how much will be paid.[18] Among the results: frustrated consumers who feel that they are considered less important than the bureaucratic process to which they are subjected.

3. An excessive amount of paperwork that escalates costs and frustrates doctors, nurses, and other medical practitioners by draining away large chunks of their time from practicing medicine.

4. The emergence of large, unnecessary costs attributable to misallocations of medical resources, overuse, fraud, and simple gaming of the system, among other reasons.

Three very different efforts to identify these issues more precisely shed light on the nature and extent of the problem. The *New York Times* conducted a year-long investigation of Medicaid in New York that produced a stunning set of revelations of fraud and abuse of the system.[19] Examples include a dentist who claimed, and was paid for, as many as 991 procedures a day; van services for patients who cannot walk used routinely by those who can at an unjustified cost estimated at $200 million per year; and a nursing home operator who received $1.5 million in salary and profit in the same year that he was fired for neglecting the residents of the home. The authors of the investigation summarized: "The program has been misspending billions of dollars annually because of fraud, waste and profiteering. A computer analysis of several million records obtained under the state Freedom of Information Law revealed numerous indications of fraud and abuse that the state had never looked into." The retired chief state investigator of Medicaid fraud and abuse in New York City, James Mehmet, who retired in 2001, believed that fraudulent claims made up at least 10 percent of state Medicaid dollars, while 20 or 30 percent more were siphoned off by what was termed "abuse," or unnecessary spending that might not be criminal. Mr. Mehmet concluded that "about 40 percent of all claims are questionable."[20]

Another sign of unnecessary costs is the vast difference in Medicaid spending between states. In 2004, New York had 4.6 million people enrolled in the system and $41.6 billion in Medicaid spending. By contrast, California had 10 million people enrolled and $31 billion in Medicaid spending. The per-enrollee cost is $9,435 in New York compared with $3,100 in California.

Dramatic regional differences in spending occur not only in the Medicaid program but also in Medicare. John Wennberg and associates at Dartmouth Medical School conducted a study focusing on the results of these differences in the late 1990s, and their findings are detailed and nuanced.[21] They identified large differences in Medicare spending between comparable groups of sixty-five-year-olds living in Miami and Minneapolis ($8,414 versus $3,341 per enrollee, respectively) and concluded that higher spending did not lead to more effective care. They attributed this result to supply-induced, as distinct from need-induced, spending. The Dartmouth group found, for example, that cardiac bypass surgery rates were "strongly correlated with the numbers of per capita cardiac catheterization labs in the regions, but not with illness rates as measured by the incidence of heart attacks in the region." Their conclusions point to potential gains from greater use of proved treatments as well as from the elimination of unnecessary measures: "The gains from improving the quality of care are too large to be ignored. They include preventing and reducing morbidity and saving lives and money. The gains from reducing disparities in Medicare spending are also too large to be ignored. The goals are not unreasonable; after all, large metropolitan areas such as Minneapolis and Portland are getting along just fine with relatively modest Medicare expenditures."[22]

Still another study that compared the relative use of health care with outcomes arrived at similar conclusions. From 1971 to 1982, RAND, a California think tank, conducted a detailed health insurance experiment that examined the effect of varying coinsurance rates and deductibles on health care expenditures and outcomes. The study, the most comprehensive of its kind, tracked 1,400 families for three years and 600 families for five years. The health of each individual in the experiment was assessed through a comprehensive battery of tests to gauge physical, mental, social, and general health. Coinsurance rates ranged from 0 to 95 percent. Deductibles, the amount the insured must pay before the insurer begins to cover expenses, ranged from 5 to 15 percent of family income up to a maximum of $1,000.

Unsurprisingly, the RAND study found that higher deductibles and higher coinsurance rates led to less frequent use of the health care system and reduced expenditures on health care. For example, a 25 percent coinsurance rate, as compared with free access, led to a 19 percent reduction in expenditures. The conclusion was one of basic economics, even in the area of health care: Higher prices lead to more careful consideration of alternatives and to lower consumption of often unnecessary services.

What surprised many, however, was that individuals in the high-deductible, high copay insurance plans were just as healthy at the end of the study as individuals whose health care was fully paid for by their employers or by government programs. As the authors of the study put it, "Our results show that the 40 percent increase in services on the free-care plan had little or no measurable effect on health status for the average adult."[23] The only significant differences between the two groups came in the categories of dental care and hypertension (high blood pressure) among the poorest

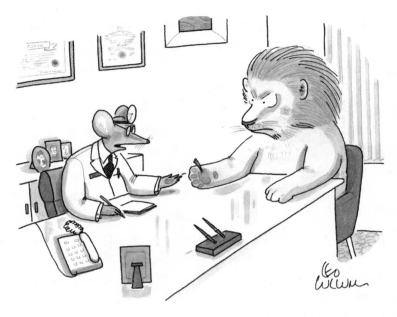

*"It is thornlike in appearance, but I need
to order a battery of tests."*

6 percent in the sample. Among the low-income individuals who had plans without dental coverage, there was a tendency to avoid visiting the dentist and therefore to develop dental problems, while low-income individuals in high-deductible plans often were unaware that they had hypertension and lived with the condition for significant periods without treatment. This problem could be eliminated simply by having individuals screened for hypertension before being enrolled in high-deductible plans.

The key result of the RAND study was that health

care consumers who were responsible for more of their health care costs through higher coinsurance rates and deductibles spent less money on health care without any adverse impact on their health.

Other studies and an abundance of anecdotal evidence all point to the conclusion that unnecessary spending on health care is rampant. For example, Dr. Arnold Milstein, the medical director of the Pacific Business Group on Health, summarized in Senate testimony the results of his work on this subject as follows: "Inefficiencies in health care delivery comprise up to 40 percent of current health care spending, and these inefficiencies can be eliminated by identification and reward of better performing physicians, hospitals, and treatment options."[24]

These conclusions are both disconcerting and encouraging: disconcerting because there are so many unnecessary costs in the system; encouraging because with an improved system there are vast opportunities to attain health outcomes that equal or surpass those produced by the current system at a substantially lower cost.

CHAPTER EIGHT

How to Improve
Health Care

WHILE EMPLOYER-PROVIDED health insurance and
the government's programs of Medicare and Medicaid
were developing as means to pay for medical care,
another health-related system was roaring along.
Scientific research and development have produced a
burgeoning array of medications, medical procedures,
and instruments, along with a growing understanding
of the basic elements of human health, all of which have
made dramatic contributions to the length and quality
of life. The following brief account of these developments includes a few suggestions on how to keep this
process rolling and puts the issues of access to the health
insurance system into reasonable perspective.

Milestones of Health Care Improvement

The discovery of penicillin in 1928 by the Scottish sci-
entist Alexander Fleming is an important landmark
in the history of biomedical research and develop-

ment. By chance, a mold had contaminated a culture of staphylococci bacteria, and Fleming observed that the bacteria surrounding the mold were disintegrating. Some substance in the mold was lethal to bacteria, and Fleming named it penicillin. Further investigation showed that penicillin was nontoxic in animals. The results intrigued Fleming, but he was unable to purify the substance or produce it in large quantities. Research stalled for almost a decade until Ernst Chain and Howard Florey, with support from the Rockefeller Foundation, took up the effort at Oxford. When they succeeded in purifying the substance, the importance of penicillin quickly became apparent to many scientists in the medical community, and research took off. In his Nobel Prize lecture in 1945, Sir Alexander Fleming said:

> Their [Chain and Florey's] results were first published in 1940 in the midst of a great war when ordinary economics are in abeyance and when production can go on regardless of cost. I had the opportunity this summer of seeing in America some of the largest penicillin factories which have been erected at enormous cost and in which the mould was growing in large tanks aerated and violently agitated. To me it was of especial interest to see how a simple observation made in a hospital bacteriological laboratory in London had eventually developed into a large industry and how what everyone at one time thought was merely one of my toys had by purification become the nearest

approach to the ideal substance for curing many of our common infections.[1]

Ernst B. Chain noted in his own Nobel lecture on March 20, 1946: "We at Oxford have been greatly handicapped in our work by lack of material. The American workers were in a more fortunate position; the Merck group alone has used up many hundred grams of pure crystalline penicillin."[2]

So what began as basic research was transformed by the realization of applicability. This realization was followed by a massive collaboration by academic scientists and a wide variety of pharmaceutical groups with substantial funding from private and public sources. The impact on the price of a dose of penicillin was dramatic: In 1940 the drug was unavailable, by July 1943 it was available at twenty dollars per dose, and by 1946 its price had been reduced to fifty-five cents per dose.

The history of the polio vaccine provides another example of stunning scientific progress. The 1954 Nobel Prize in Medicine went to John Enders, Thomas Weller, and Frederick Robbins for their development of tissue culture methods that enabled them to grow the polio virus in various types of tissue. Interestingly, penicillin played an important role in the development of the polio vaccine, for it was incorporated into the polio culture fluid to prevent the growth of bacteria, thus making it possible to grow large quantities of the polio virus on a production scale. Jonas Salk, an immunologist, figured out how to inactivate, or kill, the polio virus grown in such tissue cultures and then use it to immunize people. Clinical trials began in 1954, and on April 12, 1955, the drug was declared safe and effective. The result: a world in which polio has been almost eradicated.

More recently, research on recombinant DNA and the implementation of genetic engineering emerged from basic research by Nobel laureate Paul Berg at Stanford University and from further elaboration on that technology by two San Francisco Bay Area scientists, Stanley Cohen, a professor of medicine at Stanford, and Herbert Boyer, a biochemist at UC–San Francisco. By 1973, recombinant DNA technology had allowed Cohen and Boyer to clone genetically engineered DNA molecules in foreign cells. Their basic research, funded by the National Institutes of Health (NIH), resulted in the development of blockbuster drugs that can be mass-produced. An example is the use of human insulin to treat diabetes, a dramatic improvement in safety and effectiveness over the pig insulin treatment previously used.

Scientists are eradicating or reducing the severity of many other diseases. Open-heart surgery and pacemakers routinely prolong many productive lives. George Shultz walks comfortably on a new knee, as do many others with artificial knees and hips. X-rays, CT scans, PET scans, and MRIs have emerged as powerful diagnostic tools that often take the place of intrusive surgery. The technology that made the MRI possible grew out of research in physics and a variety of other disciplines, and the research pipeline is full of other exciting developments. For example, the mapping of the human genome is gradually leading to the ability to produce medications keyed to individual needs. Research on the use of stem cells, though controversial in some forms, gives every indication of great promise.

So a pattern has emerged: Basic research is the key that turns the lock. Academic science drives and engages scientists in the corporate world, which is oriented toward the development of useful commercial products. Government and philanthropic funding is essential for continued progress in the basic sciences, while corporate investments spur scientific projects with potential value in the marketplace.

Research also continues to teach us how personal behavior and lifestyle can make a large impact on health. Epidemiological research has identified smoking as the leading cause of lung cancer, so the use of tobacco has dropped perceptibly, at least in the United States. More recently, the Veterans Administration has studied the relationship of physical activity to health. The study followed health patterns of four matched samples of people: those who were sedentary and those who walked four thousand, six thousand, or ten thousand steps a day. The effect of that physical activity was significant.[3] Benefits were seen with about thirty minutes of moderate-intensity exercise on most days of the week, which could be achieved by walking, cycling, swimming, or even doing household chores. Even that small amount of activity was associated with a 20 percent reduction in mortality. Another study that developed a measure of energy use per day observed a sample of older adults, each of whom was assigned to one of three groups according to his or her range of normal daily activity. For example, some subjects were more likely than others to climb stairs. Researchers found that adults in the group with the highest energy expenditure had one-half the mortality rate of those in the group with the lowest expenditure of energy.[4] So lifestyle makes an undeniable contribution to health. No doubt there is a dramatic difference in overall health and life expectancy between an obese, sedentary smoker and a lean, moderately active nonsmoker.

Still another example of potential improvement of health and savings in costs can come from dealing more effectively with high blood pressure. Dr. Wade Smith, a professor of neurology at UC–San Francisco, has told us that simple treatment of hypertension could cut the number of strokes in the United States in half, from 700,000 cases per year to less than 350,000. The cost savings would come to around $40 billion per year.

All these scientific advances in the United States have emerged from a loosely associated network that includes the NIH, philanthropic funding, expanding capabilities in university research laboratories, and research and development activities in the big pharmaceutical companies and the emerging biotechnology industry. Funding from all these sources has more than doubled in the last decade.[5] Perhaps even more important, the excitement generated by what has been accomplished and the anticipation of what lies ahead have attracted some of the country's best minds, whether in universities or in biotech and pharmaceutical companies. Contributions made by chemists, biologists, and physicists have been stimulated in many cases by collaboration with gifted medical practitioners. It is no accident that some of the most productive work in health-related science has been accomplished in university laboratories that are associated with hospitals.

The link between basic research and development has led to significant advances in health care, but it has also created some problems. Prior to the early 1980s, few NIH-funded basic discoveries were commercialized because most companies found it too risky to invest in expensive development efforts when they did not own the underlying patents. With the passage of the landmark Bayh-Dole Act in 1980, universities were permitted to patent inventions created in their laboratories, a development that has led to a sharp improvement in the commercialization of scientific discoveries. The challenge for university laboratories and projects funded by NIH or private donors is to keep university scientists focused on basic research, leaving commercial development to private enterprises. Since basic research is an essential ingredient for progress in the long run

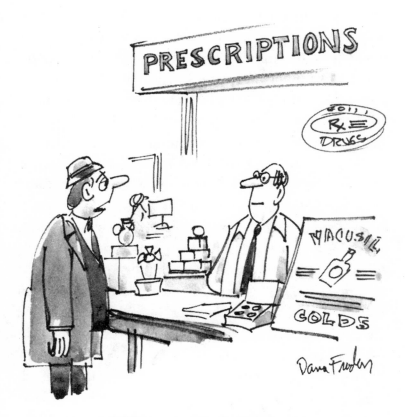

"I'll have an ounce of prevention."

and since the university setting is its natural home, arrangements for the transmission of research results into commercial applications need to be done with care. Universities and their scientists deserve to be rewarded for their efforts, but in a way that keeps them at their basic work.

The proliferation of scientific advances in the United States is also catching on around the world. Other countries—Singapore, for example—have become aware of the potential benefits of the association between academic and research institutions with commercial enterprises that profit from producing needed drugs and medical devices while employing growing numbers of workers. However, the United States leads the way. Dr. David Gratzer summarizes in his book *The Cure*: "Americans are at the forefront of this medical revolution; people from all over the world seek American medicine when they need help. And American excellence isn't confined to the hospital: When three hundred leading internists were asked to rank major medical innovations in a survey for the journal *Health Affairs*, eight of the top ten they ranked were developed, in whole or in part, in the United States."[6]

The twentieth century saw life expectancy at birth expand by nearly thirty years, in considerable part because of this research and development work. This remarkable growth in longevity is clear, but what is the monetary value of these gains? Many economists have tried to answer that question. Professor of Economics William Nordhaus, of Yale, found that if the value to individuals of gains in life expectancy (the statistical value of life) were taken into account, economic growth since 1950 would be roughly double what is currently recorded.[7] To put it another way, the increase in life expectancy since 1950 is as valuable as all other improvements, such as cars, television, iPods, and so on, combined. Research by economists Kevin Murphy and Robert Topel, professors at the University of Chicago, largely supports this conclusion and further suggests the immense value of future gains. They conclude: "Cumulative gains in life expectancy after 1900 were worth over $1.2 million to the representative American in 2000, whereas post-1970 gains added about $3.2 trillion per year to national wealth, equal to about half of GDP. Potential gains from future health improvements are also large; for example, a 1 percent reduction in cancer mortality would be worth $500 billion."[8]

From the standpoint of a healthy America and, by extension, a healthy world, a few broad conclusions can be drawn:

- Potential contributions to human health from this collaborative effort on research and development in the health area have been monumental, with continuing potential in the future. Basic research is being done mostly in universities with development work being carried out mainly in big pharmaceutical and smaller biotech companies.

- Basic research, a necessary ingredient for producing medical advances, is not motivated by or directed toward commercial objectives, so funding typically comes from private foundations or the government. In the United States most comes from the NIH. These have been among the most high-powered and productive dollars spent by the federal government, so the recent slowdown in the growth of NIH funding needs to be reexamined, perhaps by an independent group of experts. As Murphy and

Topel put it, "Our analysis suggests that the returns to basic research may be quite large, so that substantially greater expenditures may be worthwhile."[9]

- Incentives for development are also essential. Scientific research and development are time-consuming and costly, and many efforts wind up in blind alleys. When a drug is finally approved, it can usually be produced with low marginal costs, but in financing access to drugs, care must be taken to retain necessary incentives for producers.

- Tensions and difficulties certainly exist in the current system. They include the opportunity cost of delay in the use of new drugs or procedures, concerns about safety and side effects from high-powered medications or intrusive procedures, the variable pricing of drugs in different countries and the related issue of import restrictions, and the availability of low-cost drugs for HIV-AIDS patients in low-income countries.

- Despite these difficulties, a productive and energetic system has emerged in the United States and many other countries that is an essential ingredient in the improved length and quality of our lives.

CHAPTER NINE

First Steps
Toward Change

THE CURRENT U.S. health care system has many accomplishments to its credit, but it is saddled with serious problems that must be addressed. Costs, many of which are unnecessary, are on the road to levels that cannot be sustained. The health care system has evolved in a way that has produced a two-legged stool. One leg of the stool consists of providers of services, including hospitals, physicians and other practitioners, and insurance companies. Another leg of the stool is composed of those who finance health care, primarily employers and the federal and state governments. Until recently beneficiaries of the health care system had little incentive to evaluate its relative costs from the standpoint of a normal consumer. Instead, they had every incentive to use the system with little restraint because they did not bear a significant part of the costs. For the stool to stand over a prolonged period of time, the provider leg and the financier leg must be joined by a consumer leg. This process has begun, but it has a long way to go.

What does it take to make this third leg, representing the consumer, sturdy? The first step is to ensure that consumers have a significant financial stake in the system and an ability to make informed decisions about their own health care coverage. Competition among insurers is needed to lower the cost of premiums and to properly align coverage with the varying needs of those seeking insurance. This ability to choose can make the consumer an active player in the system with some degree of control. In order to be an effective participant, the consumer must have the ability to make intelligent choices through access to information about costs, quality of care, and outcomes. What is not directly available to the consumer could be available through insurance companies or other organizations. This means that careful thought must be given to ways in which to remove current inhibitions against the provision of information that were established to prevent lawsuits or the invasion of personal privacy. With empowered consumers, competitive markets for providers, and information about alternatives available to consumers, all the elements for a successful health care system—a sturdy three-legged stool—will be in place.

Can competition work as effectively in the area of health care as it does in other industries? Ample evidence exists that the answer is yes, and Michael Cannon and Michael Tanner, economists at the Cato Institute, cite numerous examples to make this point in their book *Healthy Competition*.[1] A dramatic case is the relatively recent emergence of laser eye surgery, a service for which patients pay directly and in which surgeons compete for their business. Cannon and Tanner summarize:

> Patients . . . weigh the costs and benefits of laser eye surgery, a . . . highly competitive market where prices have fallen dramatically. . . . The average price for Lasik surgery in 1999 was about $2,100 per eye. Within two years, it had fallen to less than $1,600 per eye. Many patients pay less. The price of refractive surgery dropped even more relative to overall inflation and medical inflation. Were [the numbers] to adjust for quality improvements—a driving factor behind recent price increases—it would show that average prices have fallen even more dramatically. It is also notable that these falling prices occur despite the fact that more than 80 percent of Lasik patients search for an experienced surgeon with a strong reputation, rather than just the lowest price.[2]

Against this background, what has been happening as employers and federal and state governments, the large financial players, have experienced increasing pressure? Remember, the yearly double-digit growth in the cost of health care is the source of the pressure and many of the problems in the system. Individuals can be priced out of the insurance market, and employers confronted with out-of-control health insurance costs may sharply modify the benefit structure they offer their employees or discontinue health benefits altogether, despite their tax-advantaged status. Pressure on state, city, and federal government budgets can create a sense of urgency about the need for change.

Information

If consumers are to be intelligent buyers, they must have access to information about the prices and outcomes of services they might need. Health care lags behind almost every other category of products on this score. Nevertheless, an explosion of information about diseases, treatments, prices, and outcomes seems to be under way.

Internet and health care entrepreneurs are playing a major part in bringing medical information to consumers, who currently have access to approximately twenty thousand health-related Web sites. About 80 percent of the estimated ninety-five million adult Internet users in the United States have searched for health information online.[3] Of them, 42 percent report that their medical searches had an effect on their own or someone else's health care; another 11 percent said that the information they gleaned had a major impact.[4] Physicians are increasingly turning to the Internet for help with research and diagnosis of rare conditions.[5] Patients can find Web sites for therapeutic and generic substitutes for brand-name drugs. Other sites provide links and references to local doctors and health care providers who are friendly to Health Savings Accounts (HSAs) and other types of consumer-directed health care.

Some new health care providers offer alternatives to the

traditional physician consultation. Small clinics staffed by nurse practitioners are proliferating in pharmacies and large retail stores such as Target and Wal-Mart, where no appointments are needed and information is provided along with minor treatments. Christopher Bowe, in the *New York Times* on December 6, 2007, notes that "Take Care, acquired this year by the drugstore group Walgreens, estimates it will open one clinic a day and have more than 400 by this time next year. The industry is expected to reach 5,000–10,000 retail clinics in the next few years."[6] This is a development of great importance and great potential for reducing the cost of relatively routine health care and guiding people to less expensive generic drugs. According to Dr. Jerome Grossman of Harvard's Kennedy School, clinics and similar retail activities are part of an important long-term trend in health care delivery. He notes that "there is growing evidence that a significant majority of physicians' work could be done more consistently and cost-effectively by technicians under the supervision of physicians and using advanced evidence-based decision support systems."[7]

Some health insurers, such as Aetna and Blue Cross of Minnesota, are experimenting with various transparency initiatives that would provide their customers with access to the insurance companies' actual prices and to quality data on doctors in their area.[8] This is an important step if consumers are to make intelligent, cost-effective decisions.

Other examples abound, but significant work remains

to be done. Medicare records contain vast amounts of useful price and outcome information that could be made available without revealing patients' names. Early efforts in this area show that extensive work to resolve privacy and litigation concerns is necessary before this practice becomes widespread.[9]

The emergence of information on prices and outcomes has been spurred by the empowered consumer and is a critical ingredient in improving health care. It represents an encouraging trend because it means that the consumer leg of the stool, under the pressure of mounting costs, is being strengthened by the diversion of money from providers to consumers. More payments are being made at the point of service. More consumers are gaining greater ability to choose among health providers, fueling the demand for more accurate information about prices, alternatives, and outcomes. Many problems remain, but conceptual breakthroughs, particularly with the expanding authorization of states to experiment with the structure of their Medicaid programs and the emergence of tax-advantaged Health Savings Accounts, open the way to further improvement.

Individual Health Accounts

Somehow, the U.S. body politic has gradually realized that something is missing when expenditures on health have a tax advantage only when they are made through an employer. The scope for individual choice is narrowed, insurance is lost when individuals change jobs, and care in spending is not rewarded. The result has been an evolution of the concept of tax-advantaged individual accounts that has by now come a long distance, even though the journey is not quite completed.

Authorized in 1978 by Section 125 of the Internal Revenue Code, Flexible Spending Accounts (FSAs) are designed to give employees greater control over their tax-free health care spending than they have with traditional employment-based health insurance policies.[10] Employees of companies offering FSAs can deduct a certain portion of their salaries to be set aside, tax free, in these accounts. Money in FSAs can be spent on anything from the health insurance deductible on an emergency room visit to a dental appointment to over-the-counter drugs. For example, a hypothetical worker with a salary of $50,000 may choose to send $500 to his FSA, leaving $49,500 in taxable income. This worker can spend this tax-free $500 as he sees fit, as long as it is spent on health care.

The biggest drawback of an FSA is that the money put into it is forfeited if it is not spent by the end of the year, a feature that can lead to wasteful and unusual behavior. Individuals can only guess how much money to put into their FSAs at the beginning of a year. Faced with expiring funds at the end of the year, many purchase items or services they normally would never buy, such as Botox injections, cases (rather than single bottles) of contact lens solution, designer prescription sunglasses, and unnecessary visits to the doctor.

The Health Reimbursement Account (HRA) is a logical extension of the FSA and has been on solid tax footing only since 2002. HRAs have several limitations that FSAs do not have, but they have one dramatic advantage: The balances deposited in them roll over from year to year. If an individual had $300 in an HRA on December 31, the money would still be there on January 1. With an FSA, the money would have disappeared. HRAs, however, are not portable from one job to another; an individual who switches jobs or health plans will forfeit his or her HRA balance. The HRA is similar to a company expense account in which the employee does not have full ownership of the money.

An HRA might work in the following way: A company that would normally spend $3,000 on a worker's health insurance plan might instead spend $2,500 on a higher-deductible health plan and put $500 into an HRA. The worker could spend the $500 as he or she saw fit as long as it was on health care, such as doctor visits, prescription or generic drugs, or the deductible. If the worker spent nothing on health care during the year, he or she would have $1,000 in his account in the following year (the current $500 would roll over and be combined with the $500 for next year). If the worker were to switch jobs, however, the entire HRA would disappear.

Consider two key observations:

1. People generally spend their own money more intelligently than they spend other people's money.
2. It is socially desirable to have people save for their own medical expenses.

The first point is the main idea behind FSAs and HRAs. The second notion is completely missing from FSAs and is tenuous in HRAs because the HRA balance disappears if a worker changes jobs. Growing out of work by John Goodman at the National Center for Policy Analysis, legislation in 1996 created the Medical Savings Account (MSA). The bill passed only after heated debate and was sponsored by a bipartisan group of senators led by Nancy Kassebaum and Edward Kennedy. MSAs, which were required to be coupled with a high-deductible health insurance plan, were structured like Individual Retirement Accounts. Employers could make contributions to an MSA, and that money could be spent, tax free, on health care. Balances would roll over from year to year and from job to job.

MSAs represented a conceptual breakthrough, but their success was limited by the numerous restrictions placed upon them. For example, only the self-employed or businesses with fewer than fifty employees were allowed to fund MSAs. Deposits into an MSA were limited to 65 percent of the individual deductible and 75 percent of the family deductible of the associated health plan.[11] Insurers were not eager to spend money developing products for such a limited market. Because of these drawbacks, the MSA was replaced by the Health Savings Account (HSA).

HSAs, created by the Medicare Prescription Drug Improvement and Modernization Act of 2003, were a more polished and better-constructed version of the

MSA and represented a major advance in consumer-directed health care. Proponents of HSAs have put forth several proposals to improve them and remove tax oddities that still exist, but their core concept makes them useful for many Americans.

To qualify for an HSA in 2008, an individual must have coverage under an HSA-qualified high-deductible health plan covering catastrophic—that is, high-cost—illnesses. The annual deductible must be at least $1,100 for an individual and $2,200 for a family, and the total deductible and copayments cannot exceed $5,600 for an individual and $11,200 for a family. Yearly contributions are pretax and cannot be higher than the deductible. Employers or employees can contribute, and the money in the HSA can be spent without tax on qualified medical expenses. Many suggestions have been made to improve HSAs, but in their present form they offer a widely available tax-advantaged system that allows consumers to decide on their own medical expenses and be protected from large outlays by catastrophic insurance. While HSAs are portable, the accompanying catastrophic insurance may not be.[12]

Strengthening the Consumer Leg in Medicaid and Medicare

The federal government has also taken important actions in the Medicaid field. Section 1115 of the Social Security Act enables states to apply for waivers to change their

Medicaid programs in ways that depart from general federal standards. States are applying for waivers to institute a variety of innovative programs from disease management and preventive care to the use of the HSA concept, the classification of recipients according to risk, and the use of funds for private-sector health insurance as distinct from eligibility for benefits.

The federal government's Deficit Reduction Act of 2005, estimated by the Congressional Budget Office to reduce direct Medicaid spending by $26 billion over the next ten years, expands the costs that states can require Medicaid beneficiaries to pay themselves.[13] The maximum level of these shared costs, usually in the form of copayments and deductibles, varies depending on a family's income in relation to the poverty line. A family with income above 150 percent of the federal poverty line can have more cost sharing imposed upon it than a family under 150 percent of the federal poverty line. The DRA also tightens the rules surrounding eligibility for long-term care and takes a tough stand against abuses of Medicaid through Medicaid planning, which is the spending down of assets in order to qualify for Medicaid.

Two examples of state initiatives to control cost growth and enhance the quality of service are instructive. South Carolina ranks fourth highest in state and local Medicaid spending per resident but forty-seventh highest in health outcomes, according to *Governing* magazine, a monthly publication whose primary audience is state and local government officials.[14] In Florida, 24 percent of the state's budget goes to Medicaid, and the cost of the program has grown 13 percent per year over the past six years. These states are not unique in their levels and growth rates of Medicaid spending or coverage levels. They do stand out among the states, however, in their proactive efforts to confront the problem.

Under the South Carolina Healthy Connections plan proposed by Governor Mark Sanford, every Medicaid beneficiary would receive a Personal Health Account (PHA). PHAs would be funded by the state's Medicaid program and would receive money sufficient to purchase health coverage. The amount of money in these PHAs would vary according to an individual's health history on a basis adjusted for the presumed variations in risk associated with the insured individual. For example, an older individual, who would be expected to have higher health spending, would receive more than a younger individual, and someone with diabetes would receive more than someone without diabetes because his or her expected health care costs would be higher. Risk adjustment makes insurers willing to accept patients with different risk characteristics on an equal basis because they are compensated for the risks by variations in premiums paid.

Medicaid beneficiaries could use the funds in their PHAs to purchase health coverage. Their options would include plans similar to those that employers offer their employees, such as Health Maintenance Organizations (HMOs) or Preferred Provider Organizations (PPOs).

Another option would be a catastrophic insurance policy with a high deductible, in which the PHA balance would be used in a way similar to an HSA. Whichever option is chosen, the PHA could be used for the premium, copayments, and any additional health services the enrollee might want to purchase.

Florida has also applied for a waiver under Section 1115 of the Social Security Act to reform its Medicaid system. Florida's Medicaid reform plan essentially switches Medicaid's fee-for-service system to a managed care system. Under the reform, a Florida Medicaid enrollee chooses a qualifying plan provided by a Health Maintenance Organization (HMO) or Provider Service Network (PSN), the state of Florida pays risk-adjusted premiums to the plan, and the health care plans pay for services used by the enrollee. Copayments and coinsurance costs cannot exceed those allowed under Florida's traditional Medicaid plan. Individuals may also opt out of the state Medicaid program and instead direct their Medicaid premium dollars toward a health plan sponsored by their employers.

Florida's Medicaid reform also allows for the creation of Enhanced Benefit Accounts. Money can be placed into these accounts as a reward for behavior conducive to good health, such as enrolling in a heart disease management plan, and can be used to fund other health expenditures, such as over-the-counter drugs or first-aid supplies. Funds in an Enhanced Benefit Account roll over from year to year.

Many other states have undertaken more focused Medicaid reforms through the use of Section 1115 waivers. An example is Vermont, with its Choices for Care program for elderly Medicaid beneficiaries needing long-term care. Under normal Medicaid rules, the government would pay for a senior's long-term care in a nursing home, but it would not pay for cheaper and more flexible care delivered in the patient's home. The commissioner for Vermont's Division of Disability and Aging Services called this a "crazy situation" in that "the service that people don't want and is more expensive" is guaranteed by the government while "the service people prefer and is cheaper, isn't."[15]

Vermont's Choices for Care program improves this situation by allowing Medicaid dollars to be used in more flexible ways. Instead of entering a nursing home, an elderly Medicaid beneficiary can use Medicaid dollars to pay a family member to provide him or her with home health care. This increased flexibility makes beneficiaries happier and has the potential to help the government save money.

A common trend in all these state reforms is that they move away from entitlement to services toward entitlement to a kind of voucher used to purchase services. In South Carolina, the proposed plan creates a Personal Health Account that can be used to purchase a variety of insurance plans. In Florida's program, instead of being entitled to services paid for by Medicaid, a beneficiary is entitled to a risk-adjusted amount of money that is used to purchase insurance from among several choices that meet criteria set by Florida's Medicaid program. In Vermont's program, rather than simply being entitled to nursing home care, a beneficiary is entitled to funds that can be used for long-term care in flexible ways.

Medicare is also moving in this direction through the Medicare Advantage program, an alternative to standard fee-for-service Medicare. Under Medicare Advantage, Medicare beneficiaries can enroll in a number of private-sector health plans, such as HMO plans, PPO plans, private fee-for-service plans, and various special-needs plans. The provider of the health plan receives a risk-adjusted payment from the federal government, and, in turn, the Medicare beneficiary has a private-sector health plan.

Medicare Advantage plans, which have expanded in recent years, now cover nearly seven million beneficiaries.[16] With the use of risk-adjusted payments, health insurance companies are increasingly willing to enroll not only healthy individuals but also sick Medicare recipients requiring costly care.[17] A patient with complex health problems would be very expensive to the health insurance company providing his or her coverage, but with risk adjustment, the company would receive a larger check from the government.

An interesting example of competition controlling costs and delivering quality service is the case of the Medicare prescription drug benefit. While it is a heavily

regulated form of managed competition, the drug benefit has significantly more private-sector involvement and
individual choice than traditional Medicare. Instead of a
single government plan with a single set of government-
negotiated prices, the Medicare drug benefit establishes
certain standards and then lets private-sector plans compete against one another for the business of beneficiaries.
Costs are controlled by market forces.

As it turns out, the costs of the prescription drug benefit came in far below expectations. The 2004 Social
Security trustees report estimated that the benefit would
cost $85 billion in 2006 and $93 billion by 2007. In 2006
the actual cost turned out to be just under $50 billion.
Expenditures in 2007 are now estimated to be $50 bil-
lion. Part of this difference came from slower than
expected growth in overall prescription drug prices, but
a significant portion came from higher than expected
competition among plans. Plan bids in 2006 came in
significantly below expectations, and plan bids in 2007
actually decreased 10 percent on average from 2006.[18]

The structure of the program presents two potentially large problems: adverse selection and moral hazard. Adverse selection can occur if, sick, high-cost
seniors migrate to plans with generous formularies and
bankrupt them because risk-adjusted payments are
insufficient. This would drive plans to compete only for
healthy seniors. Moral hazard can occur if, in response
to being insured, seniors begin using unnecessary prescription drugs because the drug costs have been

reduced (in some cases to zero). At this point these problems have not been overwhelming. In an analysis of the new program, the Nobel laureate in economics Daniel McFadden concludes that, "so far, the Part D program has succeeded in getting affordable prescription drugs to the senior population. . . . I think it is reasonable to say that the Part D market has performed as well as its partisans hoped, and far better than its detractors expected."[19]

Just as federal and state governments have responded to mounting Medicare and Medicaid costs by giving consumers more say about their own health care expenditures, so too have private employers. These employers often find themselves in highly competitive, internationalized markets where prices, and therefore costs, are under heavy pressure. In some cases, health care costs have risen so drastically that some employers —and particularly smaller employers—have been forced to stop offering health insurance. A further result is widespread movement away from plans that provide essentially open-ended specific benefits to plans with deductibles and copayments. In all types of plans, deductibles have been rising; many have more than doubled in the years from 1999 to 2005.[20] All these changes point to the emergence of the consumer as an empowered financial player, thereby strengthening the consumer leg of the stool.

CHAPTER TEN

Medicare, Medicaid, and Health Care Reform

THE PRESENT SYSTEM of health care in the United States must be changed, for it produces rapidly escalating costs that threaten to rise to unsustainable levels. In fact, as described in the previous chapter, significant changes and reforms have already started to take place. But the problems are large, and the actions taken to date are too small. We have a mixed system that is half private, half public, heavily bureaucratized, and uneven in its coverage. Some parts of the system are breathtakingly good, but other parts require extensive changes.

There is an emerging consensus that Americans should have universal access to quality health care. We agree. A bold vision and a well-thought-out plan of action are needed to secure an efficient, effective, affordable health care system for this country. Alternative ways to achieve this goal are presented in this chapter, along with our own set of recommendations.

One alternative, consistently rejected by the American political process, is to go the way of Europe and

Canada. Under their government-dominated systems, universal access is provided, bureaucracy reigns, rationing of health resources takes place by waiting lists, and European and Canadian patients have been known to use the United States as a safety valve.

Any appropriate U.S. alternative must meet certain goals. Drawing on points discussed in previous chapters, here are key criteria for an effective system that provides needed benefits and contains costs:

- Benefits should be attached to individuals because the U.S. labor force is mobile and employers come and go.
- Everyone should have reasonable access to benefits.
- A method of cost containment should be built into the system, with insurance companies and other providers of services subject to the pressures of competition.
- Systematic variations in the risk of health problems, such as the plain fact that risk rises with age, should be recognized.

We shall present a set of proposals that meet our basic criteria. These proposals will be best understood when placed against the background of four other ways of working toward the goals we have set out. To an important degree, we draw ideas from each of the alternatives.

The Friedman Plan

The late Milton Friedman, who won the Nobel Prize in Economics in 1976 and was certainly one of the greatest economists of the past century, set out his approach in "How to Cure Health Care," published in the winter of 2001. At the time he wrote this article, Medical Savings Accounts were new and limited; nevertheless, he saw great potential in them when combined with universal catastrophic health insurance. Friedman proposed that the current Medicare and Medicaid systems change to a system in which participants would receive a major medical insurance policy with a high deductible and a specified deposit in a health savings account. Current participants would be given the option to continue with their present arrangement or to participate in the new system. He believed this arrangement would be less expensive and bureaucratic than the current fee-for-service system and that participants would prefer such plans because of the level of choice they afford. Friedman wrote: "It would be a way to voucherize Medicare and Medicaid . . . [enabling] . . . participants to spend their own money on themselves for routine medical care and medical problems, rather than having to go through HMOs and insurance companies, while at the same time providing protection against medical catastrophes."[1] He went on to describe a more radical reform that would provide catastrophic insurance coupled with health savings accounts for every family in the United States. He also favored ending the current tax exemption of employer-based health insurance and removing "the restrictive regulations that are now imposed on medical insurance—hard to justify with universal catastrophic insurance."[2]

Friedman laid out a conceptual framework providing universal coverage that empowers consumers and focuses insurance on catastrophic risks. His call for a sweeping change in the system providing access to health care meets our criteria.

The Fuchs-Emanuel Plan

In a similar but more detailed fashion, Victor Fuchs, an emeritus professor at Stanford University who is widely considered one of the leading health economists in the country, and Ezekiel Emanuel, of the National Institutes of Health, have developed a comprehensive plan for universal health insurance through Friedman-like vouchers for all Americans.[3] Their plan would enable individuals and families to choose from several privately offered basic health insurance plans with relatively low deductibles and copayments. Individuals could pay for additional services not covered under their basic plan or upgrade to premium insurance policies with their own after-tax money.

All the basic plans would offer benefits similar to those offered by large employers today and would provide adequate coverage for most people. A government board would determine the minimum coverage of the basic plans. The vouchers would be risk adjusted so that their value would reflect the age, gender, health history, and expected use of health services by each participant. All the basic health insurance plans would offer guaranteed enrollment and renewals for all Americans.

Everyone would have a choice of plans, and everyone would have high-quality coverage.

Like Milton Friedman's concept, the Fuchs-Emanuel plan would eliminate the tax exemption for employer-provided health insurance. With the issuance of universal vouchers and the removal of tax incentives for employment-based health insurance, it is likely that employers would quickly get out of the business of providing health insurance.

Under the Fuchs-Emanuel plan, Medicaid and other means-tested government health insurance programs would be replaced immediately by universal vouchers. Because the new program would cover everyone, there would be no reason to have separate programs for low-income individuals. On the other hand, Medicare would be phased out gradually. Current participants could remain on the traditional Medicare plan for the rest of their lives, but Medicare would not accept new enrollees. In the future, those turning sixty-five would simply continue with the universal voucher health insurance program. Ultimately there would be one program, with choice within the program, for everyone.

The Fuchs-Emanuel plan for universal vouchers would be funded by a new value-added tax, essentially a dedicated national sales tax, the revenues of which would be strictly devoted to the voucher plan. The advantage of dedicating the revenue source is that it links the benefits of the program to its costs. Proposals to enhance benefits would necessitate tax rate increases, so any proposal to expand the basic plans would require a debate about whether the extra benefits from the new proposal would justify the additional costs. General revenue financing, which is currently employed for Parts B and D of Medicare, allows politicians to avoid this tough question. Benefits, such as Medicare prescription drugs, have been added without identifying where the additional funds will come from. Fuchs and Emanuel argue that tax dedication would force better decision making. We agree, but we worry that the political process will find a way around this safeguard if it wants to. We also question the feasibility of combining massive reform of the health care system with a substantial change in the tax system. Either of these is a big undertaking.

Another feature of the Fuchs-Emanuel plan would be the establishment of an independent Institute for Technology and Outcomes Assessment. It would play a key role in providing the marketplace with unbiased information about the efficacy of various treatments, the services and treatments that should be included in universal coverage, and what should be left to choice. In order to have a system that empowers consumers with choice, consumers must have unbiased information on which to base their decisions. Fuchs and Emanuel propose that one-half of 1 percent of the revenues raised to support their system of universal vouchers be directed toward funding this institute.

The Fuchs-Emanuel plan would probably be no

more expensive than the sum of our current system of employment-based health insurance (partly paid for by tax subsidies), separate programs for low-income individuals such as Medicaid, Medicare for the elderly, and emergency room treatment for the uninsured (paid for by taxpayers and the insured). But their plan would create more cost-conscious, informed consumers with a resultant pressure on costs.

Of course, employers do not provide free health insurance to their employees; wages and salaries are lowered by the compensation paid in the form of health benefits. If the Fuchs-Emanuel plan were adopted, companies would drop health coverage, but competition among employers would drive wages and salaries upward. Employers would still have to pay employees the marginal value of what they produced.

In addition, individual income tax rates could be lowered because of the elimination of Medicaid and the removal of the tax exemption for health insurance, which currently allows employers to provide part of their compensation to their employees tax free. Offsetting all this, of course, would be the burden of the new health insurance value-added tax. Therefore, taking everything into account, the cost of health care for the average American probably would be about the same as it is under the current system. However, the Fuchs-Emanuel plan would encourage greater competition and access to health information, and the government would be better able to predict and make provision for future costs by calculating the cost of vouchers.

The Cogan-Hubbard-Kessler Plan

A different approach has been put forward by economists John Cogan, Glenn Hubbard, and Daniel Kessler in *Healthy, Wealthy, and Wise: Five Steps to a Better Health Care System*.[4] In this carefully written book, the authors set out their recommendations, which are designed to increase competitiveness in the health care market, improve the quality of information available to participants in the market, and improve the capacity of consumers to exercise effective choices. We include their ideas in our own recommendations.

The President George W. Bush Plan

Still another approach was put forward by President Bush in his 2007 State of the Union address. He proposed, as have Friedman and Fuchs-Emanuel, to fix one of the federal tax code's most damaging and distorting—and most enduring—features, the tax exclusion for employer-provided health insurance.

Because health expenditures by an employer are not counted as compensation, health care purchased by the employer is not taxed, whereas health care purchased by an individual is taxed. This heavily favors health care expenditures by an employer over expenditures by an individual, and the more the employer spends, the larger the federal tax subsidy. This encourages expensive, low-deductible health plans and third-party payer systems that drive up the costs for everyone. The total value of the federal tax subsidy is now on the order of $200 billion a year.

Policy makers have long wanted to remove this tax exclusion but have considered the idea dead on arrival. Cogan, Kessler, and Hubbard write: "The best way to reverse this trend [toward low-deductible insurance] would be to revoke the tax preference. Unfortunately, as experience from the tax-reform debates of the 1980s showed, this solution appears politically infeasible."[5] Sometimes what appears infeasible actually may be possible. In an innovative way, President Bush has proposed a palatable replacement for the tax exclusion that is far more efficient economically.

The president's proposal removes the tax exclusion from employment-based health expenditures while moving the tax subsidy to individuals. Specifically, his proposal would create a standard deduction for having health insurance and end the tax exclusion for employer-provided health insurance. The deduction would total $7,500 for an individual and $15,000 for a family. Importantly, the size of the deduction would depend not on the cost of the health insurance purchased but rather on demonstration that a suitable purchase had been made. An individual would get the same

$7,500 deduction if he or she had a $10,000 health insurance plan with no deductibles or a $3,000 health insurance plan with high deductibles. An individual who wanted an expensive, low-deductible plan could still get one, but the decision would no longer be distorted by the tax code. To save money, consumers would likely opt for plans with higher deductibles and coinsurance. Health insurance would begin to resemble more closely all other types of insurance, and consumers would have a greater stake in the game.

The population in the two lowest income quintiles pays no income tax and therefore would not be able to use the deduction. If the president's proposal were enacted, it would almost surely be accompanied by an equalizing tax credit for those who pay no taxes, provided on evidence of the purchase of suitable insurance. If this were done, then a wide swath of the U.S. population would be in control of purchasing their health insurance. The result would be something akin to the universal voucher system proposed by Friedman and Fuchs and Emanuel, as outlined above.

The president's proposal is estimated to be revenue neutral with some shift in the overall benefit of the federal tax subsidy from those with the most generous insurance policies to those with more standard policies. If his proposal is adopted, we shall applaud and adjust our recommendations so as to be in tune with the sharply different systems that would emerge.

An Alternative, Incremental Approach

The Fuchs-Emanuel and Friedman plans have many desirable features, as does the president's latest proposal, but they are clearly radical departures from the current system. We admire the combination of universal coverage, government-financed but privately and competitively provided health insurance, linkage of benefits to costs, and advocacy of improved information available to consumers. However, we are not convinced that it is possible to implement such a plan in one step. As an alternative, we propose, therefore, an incremental approach that would move major elements of the health care system in the same directions as those advocated by Milton Friedman and Fuchs and Emanuel.

The Shultz-Shoven set of health initiatives has several components. Unlike Fuchs and Emanuel, we do not propose replacing Medicare and Medicaid completely, nor would we suggest replacing the U.S. system of employment-based health insurance. Instead, we seek to modernize and significantly reform Medicare and Medicaid, improve employer-sponsored health plans, and ensure that those who do not have access to such plans will still be able to obtain affordable major health insurance. We advocate that all Americans have access to strengthened Health Savings Accounts and a more competitive health insurance environment.

The First Step

Health Savings Accounts, enabling individuals to save for their own potential health costs with before-tax dollars and combined with a catastrophic health insurance policy, are now available and are attracting increasing numbers of Americans. Health plans that include HSAs account for a small but rapidly growing segment of the insured population. Approximately five million individuals, many of whom were previously uninsured, are enrolled in HSAs through their employers or individually.[6] Now is the time to enhance the quality of Health Savings Accounts in ways that make them more accessible and useful. Here are four suggestions that have been endorsed by many scholars, health care practitioners, and politicians, including President George W. Bush:

1. Provide the same tax advantages for any individual who purchases an HSA as are now provided when an employer purchases an HSA for an individual. There should be no discrimination against individual initiative and the self-employed.

2. Allow the use of risk adjustment so that individuals with identifiable health problems can contribute, or their employers can contribute for them, larger amounts into their HSAs.

3. Make any out-of-pocket health care expenses tax deductible for those with fully funded HSAs.

4. Require that all HSAs, including related high-deductible catastrophic insurance policies, be portable, whether or not they were purchased for employees by their employ-

ers. A related move would make it possible for individuals to purchase portable HSAs from health insurers. As each HSA is linked to a catastrophic health insurance plan, a national market would be created for such insurance.

These changes in HSAs would make them more useful and more affordable for low-income individuals. They would also make HSAs more likely to be used by employers, units of government, or self-employed individuals looking for a way to provide health care benefits with reasonably predictable costs.

The second reform that would benefit all Americans is the establishment of a more competitive environment for health insurance, thereby making it less costly and more suitable for varying individual needs. The insurance industry is of central importance to the cost, quality, and accessibility of health care. Insurance costs have grown dramatically and continue to rise, but this is not simply a reflection of health costs. Insurance is currently available on a state-by-state basis. Because insurers and the providers they work with have large political clout in most states, insurance laws require broad, expensive coverage that often goes far beyond what most individuals need or want. Devon Herrick, an economist at the National Center for Policy Analysis, reports:

> The Commonwealth Fund and e-HealthInsurance.com compared the prices of policies in seven states with varying degrees of regulation. The policies had similar coverage and a deductible of about $500. A 25-year-old male in good health could pur-

chase a policy for $960 a year in Kentucky. That policy would cost about $5,880 in New Jersey. A similar policy available in Kansas for about $1,548 costs $5,172 in New York State. A policy priced at $1,692 in Iowa and $2,664 in Washington State would cost $4,032 in Massachusetts. The difference in premiums is mainly due to state regulations rather than variation in health care costs.[7]

Parallel bills to allow insurance to be written on a national basis have been introduced in the House of Representatives and in the Senate. If these bills pass, competition will most likely lead insurance companies to offer insurance with varying coverage so that a consumer can buy only the needed coverage, thus making it less expensive. When combined with the right of insurers to sell portable HSAs, including the required catastrophic coverage, these changes would lead to marked improvements in the health care system.

In addition to these improvements, Medicare and Medicaid must be reformed. The escalating costs and solvency of these programs are tough problems to fix. The costs depend not only on the numbers of eligible participants but, more important, on their future health status, the medical technologies available, and the incentives given to participants to consume health care efficiently and effectively. Improvements must be made to these programs and their financial outlook, concentrating first on Medicare while recognizing that some of the ideas that will improve Medicare will also be applicable to Medicaid. We shall first suggest the outline of a modernized Medicare system that maintains and improves the safety net feature of the existing program while enhancing its progressivity and efficiency.

Improve Medicare

The long-term necessity of reforming Medicare stems from its runaway costs and evidence that waste and inefficiency account for a significant portion of its expenses. Medicare costs have increased dramatically in the past forty years, not only in absolute terms but also relative to other prices, wages, and the aggregate size of the economy itself. There is no sign of a slowdown in the growth of Medicare costs. Eventually, however, unless these costs are curtailed, Medicare—and Medicaid, its companion program—will completely swamp the federal budget and the economy as a whole. It is not just the government's budget that will be unable to sustain the current structure of Medicare; the budgets of the elderly will not be able to handle it either. Medicare reform is essential for long-term solvency.

What are the keys to a comprehensive solution for this looming problem? Much can be done to make the system more efficient. Benefits can be restructured to reduce waste and improve efficiency. A modernized system could produce better health outcomes for less money than does the current design. The innovation and efficiency that accompany competitive markets are needed, as are better-informed consumers who have meaningful choices. Competition is needed so that health care providers who fail to offer high-quality products at reasonable prices are replaced in the market by providers that can. The safety net for low-income individuals must be preserved and even strengthened. A high-quality Medicare program must be designed that significantly reduces the strain on the federal budget. Medicare can be better and cheaper at the same time that it is progressive and compassionate.

How can all these things be accomplished? We come to the same conclusion as that reached by Milton Friedman, Victor Fuchs, and Ezekiel Emanuel: The best solution is a carefully designed Medicare voucher program that takes advantage of a more competitive market for insurance. As included in our ideas for Social Security reform and the transition proposed by Fuchs and Emanuel, those already receiving Medicare benefits would not be moved to the new system, although they could accept the changes if they so desired.

A voucher system would grant each eligible Medicare participant an amount of money with which to purchase comprehensive health insurance. There would be a menu of insurance options including HMOs, such as Kaiser and HealthNet, and HSAs combined with catastrophic insurance. All these plans would compete for participants. The full benefits of competition would thus be brought to the health care field.

The dollar value of the vouchers would differ

depending on a participant's age, gender, and health status, determined from previous medical records. As discussed earlier, the purpose of adjusting the value of the vouchers to health status, commonly called risk adjusting, is to avoid the problem of insurance companies attempting to enroll only the healthiest Medicare participants. Ideally, after risk adjustments, all Medicare participants, regardless of their health status, would be equally attractive customers for health insurance companies. And insurance companies could be justifiably required to take all comers. Already, Medicare Advantage plans are using the risk adjustment concept and insurers are responding aggressively, as pointed out in the previous chapter.

We recognize that risk adjustment calls for careful administration so as to avoid the problem of people cultivating risk. The more the system sticks to objective factors, the less likely is widespread gaming of the system.

The value of Medicare vouchers could also reflect the participant's earnings history. Participants whose average lifetime earnings place them in the lowest thirtieth percentile would receive the full value of their age, gender, and health-adjusted vouchers. This would permit Medicare participants with relatively low lifetime earnings to choose among alternative health insurers offering comprehensive plans with low deductibles and copayments. Under this plan, the out-of-pocket health care expenses for those in the lowest thirtieth percentile of lifetime earnings would be less than or equal to what they are under the current Medicare system.

On the other hand, those in the top twentieth percentile of lifetime earnings would receive vouchers, adjusted by age, gender, and health status, in amounts just sufficient to purchase catastrophic care insurance policies. All would be allowed to supplement the value of their Medicare grants with their own resources, as in the purchase of tax-advantaged HSAs. A schedule of voucher adjustments based on lifetime earnings would create a sliding scale from those with low lifetime earnings, who would have no reductions, to those with high lifetime earnings, who would face significant reductions.

The lifetime earnings reductions are a type of means testing for Medicare that serves two purposes. The first is to help contain the total costs of Medicare by asking those who are financially able to do so to bear a larger portion of the costs for their own health care while making sure that low-income individuals have an adequate level of Medicare benefits.

The second purpose of lifetime earnings adjustments is to preserve the incentives to save and invest in the economy. The reductions do not depend on either the wealth or income of Medicare participants. Consider, for example, two individuals with the same history of earnings, one a systematic saver and the other a big spender. In retirement, the saver is relatively wealthy with a high income whereas the spender gets by on Social Security and a much lower income. Both individuals would face the same lifetime earnings adjustment to their Medicare vouchers. The advantage of this system of means testing is that it does not discourage saving (or working, for that matter). We label this form of lifetime earnings adjustments "smart means testing."

We like the Fuchs-Emanuel proposal for establishing a dedicated revenue source for Medicare, although we recognize how adept the political process is at finding ways around restrictions. Of course, Part A has a dedicated revenue source with its 2.9 percent payroll tax. Our Medicare voucher system would merge all of Medicare's parts (A, B, C, and D) and fund them with the current payroll tax and within a commitment to a balanced federal budget at full employment. This is a way to establish the accountability advantages of tax dedication without introducing a whole new value-added tax system, as proposed by Fuchs and Emanuel.

The age of eligibility for Medicare need not be changed, although a reassessment might be appropriate at some point if life expectancies continue to march upward. Once eligible for Medicare, an individual would receive a health insurance voucher whether or not he or she was still working. This is a significant change relative to the current Medicare practice of acting as the secondary payer for a worker who receives employee health benefits from an employer with twenty or more employees. The proposed change would encourage firms to hire such individuals. Instead of being burdened with the entire health insurance cost for elderly workers, firms would find that the bulk of these costs would be provided for by Medicare vouchers.

Out-of-pocket deductibles, copayments, and the money to supplement Medicare vouchers all could come from HSAs. The extension of such accounts would promote saving among the elderly as well as among working Americans. Pretax dollars could be accumulated in tax-sheltered investment accounts and withdrawn, tax free, for out-of-pocket medical expenses and health insurance costs. Not only could the money be saved for future use, but also unspent funds could be bequeathed to one's heirs. Because they would be using their own money, people would be encouraged to be prudent when making their health care spending decisions.

The lifetime earnings–adjusted vouchers would work well for the vast majority of Medicare participants. Nonetheless, some people would fall through the safety net. For instance, an individual who had high lifetime earnings might fall into a lower-income category because of unfortunate circumstances or unavoidable costs, such as the need to provide long-term care for aging parents. In such a case, the proposed lifetime earnings–adjusted vouchers would provide only catastrophic health insurance on the mistaken assumption that such an individual would be able to supplement the voucher with personal resources. This is exactly the type of circumstance in which Medicaid comes to the rescue, because it provides a second safety net for those with very low incomes and wealth. Medicaid coverage differs by states, but its minimum benefits would be similar to the comprehensive coverage of Medicare for those with low lifetime earnings. This would retain and strengthen the safety net provided by Medicaid.

The Medicare vouchers program would permit the government to bring future costs of the system under control in several ways. First, efficiency would be enhanced because insurance providers would have to compete with one another for business. Even those participants in the bottom thirtieth percentile of lifetime earners would be involved in the program, structured to give them an element of choice. Second, those above the lowest-income group would be spending more of their own money and therefore monitoring the value-for-money balance more carefully. Third, the vouchers would convert the government's obligation from one of medical services to one of calculable cash payments.

Almost everyone who has analyzed the future of Medicare has concluded that the current practice of providing its participants with all desired health treatments regardless of cost cannot be maintained for long. Inevitably, some form of rationing or cost-effectiveness calculation will be introduced. The private market almost always makes better rationing decisions than do government bureaucrats. The best way to ration is through the marketplace, from the joint decisions of insurance companies in the design of their alternative policies to the choices made by households among the plans offered. Health care would be rationed in a manner similar to food: People would exercise choice, and those in the lowest-income group would receive assistance, just as food stamps are allocated to the needy.

Improve Medicaid

The advantages of competition in the presence of informed consumers extends to Medicaid as well as to Medicare. The traditional Medicaid system, in which eligibility carries entitlement to a range of services, has come under intense pressure as extensive fraud and misuse have damaged the system and costs have escalated rapidly. All state governments have become concerned about the impact on their budgets of the virtually runaway costs of Medicaid. The result has been an accelerating number of changes by states that obtain waivers under Section 1115 of the Social Security Act. The general trend of state governments shows a movement in the direction of small copayments and deductibles and the use of insurance or health plan vehicles that limit state costs and require Medicaid recipients to contribute more for the services they receive.

The structure of the current system of Medicaid actually discourages people from working. Eligibility depends on income and wealth and varies widely by state and by the medical condition of the recipient. The average annual benefit for a family of four is approximately $12,000, a large number reflecting the fact that a small percentage of families have extremely large health costs. What that means is that an extra burst of work for which someone is paid, say, $1,000, might push that individual above the eligibility line, causing him or her to lose a much larger amount of money. The impact on the desire to work is obvious: There is no incentive to work more if the result is less income. This suggests that one of the many necessary and desirable changes that should be made is the removal of this notch, which is a powerful disincentive to work.

Efforts to reform welfare confronted the same problem, but in that case the eligibility was for money. The solution was to disregard an initial amount of additional earnings and then phase out benefits as earnings increased further. That removed the notch and ensured that as an individual earned money, he or she would always stay ahead of the game.

A further evolution of what is already taking place in the Medicaid waiver system could make it possible to deal with this problem while also enhancing consumer involvement in the costs. Health Savings Accounts contain money, after all, but that money is devoted specifically to health. Suppose the Medicaid system gave those below the poverty line a fully funded HSA. Recipients would then have catastrophic insurance with a deductible and an amount of money that could be spent, no doubt in some prescribed way, on health costs. Unspent money would stay in the individual's account.

As a Medicaid recipient went to work and earned pay that would put him or her above the poverty line, the funding of the HSA would be gradually reduced. If the household income level reached twice the poverty line, the only remaining Medicaid benefit would be catastrophic insurance, with the family being responsible for funding the HSA. Further income increases would reduce the subsidy to the catastrophic insurance. The big change is that it always would be in the interest of the family to work harder and earn more money.

The HSA plus major medical insurance might be one of the options offered to recipients of Medicaid. As with Medicare, we advocate that participants be encouraged to choose from a menu of quality insurance options. Medicaid participants would have the same risk-adjusted voucher system as Medicare enrollees. Those at the lowest income levels could obtain a good, comprehensive health plan with little or no out-of-pocket money. They would have choice. As their incomes increased, the subsidy of their Medicaid policies would be gradually reduced.

The voucher-style Medicaid program that we are proposing would cover more people than does the current Medicaid program. Today those just above the income limits are unable to obtain Medicaid health insurance. With our proposal, those above the existing limits would still receive some Medicaid assistance.

As with Medicare, funding for Medicaid could be derived from a commitment to a balance in the federal budget at full employment. But enhancements to these programs should not be paid for out of general revenues of the federal government beyond the slice identified. It has proved too easy to ignore the fact that general revenues will be increasingly scarce in the future. Better decisions will be made about the scale of both Medicaid and Medicare if they are funded from identifiable tax sources.

We think the first step toward comprehensive health insurance reform is to empower Medicare and Medicaid participants with choice and to improve the information available to them for informed decision making.

We stop short of the full Fuchs-Emanuel and Friedman approaches to health insurance for those who are not elderly or in the lowest income brackets. We support the Fuchs-Emanuel idea of an independent Institute for Technology and Outcomes Assessment. Such an institute can develop information on prices and outcomes and identify and publicize best practices and new developments. We think that it is too soon to abandon completely the employment-based health insurance system that is the backbone of today's health delivery system. Employers are moving toward offering consumers a choice of plans, employees are rapidly adopting Health Savings Accounts, and the increased use of copayments and deductibles means that consumers are spending more of their own money.

We think that it is wise to follow along with these trends as they move toward other necessary changes. We have already listed ways that HSAs can be strengthened. They should be made more widely available, restrictions on their availability should be eased, and they should be extended to those who do not have employer-based health coverage. Health insurance markets and regulations should be national, not statewide. Catastrophic health insurance should be universally available so that all Americans can protect themselves from the unexpected expenses of big-ticket health events.

Our overall plan, as summarized in table 10.1, is to modernize radically Medicare and Medicaid, introducing more choice, better information, and smart means testing. We think that costs can be brought under control by providing a specified amount of money for health care rather than an open-ended set of services and by empowering consumers to choose among health care options, just as they make selections in other realms, such as food and housing. Markets that function well make efficient rationing decisions, so they do not experience the kind of affordability crises that health care now faces. We propose to extend this efficiency to our health care programs.

The Opportunities Ahead

The health care system established in the last half of the twentieth century provided access to medical services for many Americans who otherwise would have had great difficulty obtaining adequate care. As discussed in chapter 7, the structure of that system produced a stool with only two legs, one of providers and one of financiers. That system led to large unwarranted and unnecessary costs, fraud, and inefficiency on a broad scale. As these costs mounted, they made the system less and less affordable. Employers under competitive pressures and governments under budgetary pressures have reacted in a wide variety of ways. They have taken steps that, in effect, are building a consumer leg for the stool. Suggestions made here would strengthen that leg and afford the possibility of an improved health system. Competition would rid the system of much of the waste and misallocation of resources described in chapter 7. Universal access would be available to all Americans and would be built, in a sense, from the bottom up, the American way, as distinct from a system of universal coverage built from the top down and administered by a bureaucracy in the European way.

The ingredients are already in place. The Medicaid system, as rearranged in the way recommended here, would provide the resources needed for everyone below a poverty-like band drawn by the states. The Medicare system already provides for almost all who are sixty-five and older. If the coverage were in the form of funds, as we recommend, then resources would be in the hands of consumers. If reasonable costs could be calculated, there is every reason to believe that employment-based insurance, particularly in the form of high-deductible health plans and HSAs, would become virtually universal. In addition, revised HSAs could be offered at a reasonable cost to the self-employed. Others who may fall between the cracks of these different systems would be much more inclined to provide for themselves if HSAs were readily accessible and if insurance suited to their needs were available at a reasonable price. The ample funds already allocated within the present multifaceted health finance system would go to individuals who are becoming increasingly sophisticated consumers as they are provided with the information they need.

Health care affects each of us in a very personal way. We expect basic medical services to be broadly available. This objective can be achieved by changing the structure of the present health care system. With an improved structure in place, costs can be contained, and the health needs of all Americans can be adequately served.

Table 10.1 Summary of the Shultz-Shoven Health Initiatives

Private system	• Encourage national, rather than state, markets in health insurance, thereby promoting competition, putting downward pressure on costs, and providing reasonable choices of covered services.
	• Promote enhanced consumer information about health service prices and quality. Medicare records on the quality of hospitals and health service providers and the effectiveness of alternative treatments should be made public while the privacy of individuals is protected.
	• Strengthen the incentives for company-sponsored HSAs and accompanying catastrophic insurance by making them portable across employers and permitting tax-deductible health spending for those who have fully participated in an HSA program.
	• Make tax-advantaged HSAs and relatively low-cost catastrophic insurance available to all those who do not have employer-sponsored plans.
Medicare	• Provide risk-adjusted vouchers.
	• Offer consumer choice among plans (Kaiser-style HMO plans, high-deductible catastrophic insurance plus HSAs, and traditional Blue Cross–type plans).
	• Use smart means testing: Value of vouchers would depend on lifetime labor earnings (AIME).
	• Ensure gradual transition: Existing Medicare participants would be allowed to stay with traditional coverage.
	• Finance with dedicated taxes, thereby promoting cost effectiveness.
Medicaid	• Provide risk-adjusted vouchers.
	• Continue to allow states to experiment with structure.
	• Offer consumers choices, including HSAs with catastrophic insurance.
	• Provide increased coverage: Replace eligibility notch with phased reduction of the value of vouchers.
	• Finance federal support with dedicated taxes, thereby promoting cost-effectiveness.

CHAPTER ELEVEN

Conclusions

THE UNITED STATES is a country that has been blessed in a great variety of ways. Its citizens are healthier than at any time in the past, and, as a consequence, they are living longer than ever before. The U.S. economy is strong, creative, and productive. Too often this success is ignored and a gloomy picture is painted, largely because of forecasts of coming catastrophe. Projections of the costs of U.S. programs to provide income for the elderly through Social Security and insurance for access to the health care system uniformly carry numbers that reach into the stratosphere and are incompatible with a well-functioning economy. Such costs cannot be sustained.

These projections are useful because they reveal a scenario that cannot be allowed to materialize. They also show that the only workable response to prevent a crisis is to adjust the programs rather than simply appropriate more money. Alternative methods to accomplish the objectives of the Social Security and health care programs must be examined, debated, and implemented as soon as possible. The costs of transition from the present structure of the programs to an alternative that makes fiscal sense are inevitable, but the sooner programs are changed and put on a solvent, sustainable basis, the more controllable the transition costs will be and the more confidently citizens can plan for their future.

What guidelines should be followed when we consider the future of U.S. entitlement programs? Here are ten commandments for successful reforms:

1. Remember the pie test. Entitlements divide the GDP pie. The bigger the pie, the easier it is to make divisions. Any proposal that weakens GDP fails the pie test.

2. Deliver benefits to individuals rather than to institutions because flexibility of the labor force and the dynamic nature of private employment are bound to be characteristics of the future.

3. Increase incentives to raise labor force participation and eliminate features of the systems that discourage participation. These actions will enlarge the pie.

4. Favor reforms that have a positive impact on the personal saving rate.

5. In light of the ten-to-one ratio between the after-tax income of the top 20 percent of households and the bottom 20 percent, design reforms to create a reasonable safety net for low-income earners in their later years.

6. Identify ways to enhance the connection between what an individual pays in to what he or she receives from the Social Security system. Private accounts can help attain this goal.

7. Consider proposals to accompany reforms with any form of tax rate increase only with great reluctance and only when the added revenue has a clear use and will produce benefits that outweigh the drag on the economy from the tax rate increase.

8. Look for ways to force the political process to examine the costs of any proposed increase and identify the source of the offsetting revenue.

9. Whenever possible, make use of competitive market forces to discipline costs and to allow individuals to design programs that fit their needs.

10. Ensure that research and development systems that contribute to better health and increased longevity are supported in a way that allows those systems to flourish.

Bake a Big Pie: The Gross Domestic Product

The first step is to recognize that the gross domestic product—the pie—will have to be divided among the generations and among people with differing needs for access to the health care system. From that realization, it follows that the pie must be made as big as possible and the productivity of workers must continue to rise so that it can keep expanding.

The strength of the U.S. economy was described in chapter 1. For the past quarter century, the economy has grown strongly, inflation has been kept under control, and recessions have been mild and rare.

Certain features of the U.S. economy stand out:

- There is great flexibility. Change is constantly under way in labor markets, and new companies are continually springing up in large numbers, with many succeeding and almost as many failing to make the grade.

- Large companies that become uncompetitive shrink or disappear. Others, newly competitive and innovative, prosper. Joseph Schumpeter's description of the process of creative destruction seems to be at work and has had positive results.[1]

- Flexibility and competitiveness are connected to the relative openness of the U.S. economy, as the importance of international trade has grown steadily over the last half century.

- New ventures, products, and ideas are coming onstream, research and development activities are strong, and venture capitalists are looking for creativity and innovation.

- The low saving rate means that a significant portion of investment in the U.S. economy comes from abroad. In the future, as the need grows for sources of funds to support the growing proportion of elderly people in the population, the income stream from foreign-held assets will not be flowing into American hands. A rise in the saving rate can mitigate that problem. Recommended measures include ending federal dissaving, improving and expanding 401(k) and IRA accounts, creating personal accounts within the Social Security system, and expanding Health Savings Accounts.

- Income inequality among Americans is another emerging issue that must be confronted. The phenomenon is real, but the reasons for it are unclear. In any case, this inequality means that as changes are made in the design of Social

Security and the health care systems, special attention must be given to those in the lower levels of income distribution.

Beyond nourishing the positive characteristics of the U.S. economy and addressing its problems, there is a clear need to enhance participation in the labor force. Participation rates among Americans aged fifty and up have been falling over the past forty years, highlighting the importance of examining incentives and disincentives to work. A number of important possible changes, identified in chapter 3, could help build up participation in the labor force.

- The important analysis made by the Nobel laureate Edward Prescott, discussed in chapter 1, bears on this issue. Prescott found a negative correlation between tax rates and labor supply through his analysis of cross-country comparisons. Countries with high tax rates have relatively low work effort. Clearly, the broad decline in marginal tax rates in the United States that began in the Kennedy administration has helped maintain labor force participation. Many other steps could be taken to enhance participation.

- Employers would be encouraged to hire older workers and the incentive to work would be increased if Social Security taxes were considered paid up after forty years, for example. This practice is commonly offered by private insurers.

- Social Security benefits are now calculated on the basis of the highest thirty-five years of earnings. Earnings in other years are taxed, but they often deliver no additional Social Security benefits. We advocate counting at least forty years of work toward Social Security benefits.

- Social Security benefits become taxable when an individual earns even a modest income. At a certain level of income, this results in a marginal rate of taxation on income of around 46 percent. This is a much higher rate than Bill Gates or almost anyone else pays. Why discriminate against older workers?

- The Social Security system currently creates disincentives for long careers by the way it handles progressivity. A simple revenue-neutral change in the benefit formula could maintain the better deal given to lifetime low-income individuals but allow Social Security to distinguish them from high-income individuals who have short careers.

- The Medicare system is arranged so that if an employee is covered by a private plan, Medicare is the secondary payer. If, on the other hand, Medicare became the primary payer, older workers would become more attractive to employers and might well command better compensation.

- The Medicaid system can discourage low-income individuals from working. If their pay increases and puts them even slightly above the poverty line, they become ineligible for health benefits, which are often worth more than their extra income. The resulting notch creates a massive disincentive to work. Potential changes in Medicaid have been identified that could make it possible to ameliorate this situation.

Income for the Elderly

People instinctively think about and try to make provisions for their elderly years. Public policy should be designed to provide reasonable incentives for individuals to take care of themselves and to make it as easy as possible to do so. However, some people are more successful than others, so it is also important to create a safety net for everyone.

Chapter 4 traces the trends in employer-provided pension plans, and the conclusion is clear: Plans that provide defined benefits to retired workers are rapidly giving way to plans that allow for defined contributions. These contributions are invested and can be converted into annuities at retirement. This shift from defined benefits to defined contributions changes the structure of risks. With defined contributions, employers can reduce their risks because they can calculate costs with certainty. This change is not necessarily adverse for their employees. Recent spectacular bankruptcies show that the risk of default on defined benefit pension obligations is real and more widespread than was assumed earlier. Under the defined contribution system, employees own their plans, so movement from one employer to another does not jeopardize their pension rights. There is, of course, the risk of uncertain rates of return on investments, but if history is any guide, sensible investment programs produce reasonably stable results over extended periods of time.

Recent legislation allowing automatic enrollment in 401(k) plans makes it easier to increase the amount of money that employers or employees put into the plans.[2] This legislation also takes steps to provide individuals with improved counseling geared to guide them into reasonably high-performing investments.

Social Security has helped generations of elderly people live comfortably. In fact, the poverty rate among the elderly is lower than among nonelderly Americans, a dramatic shift from the period before Social Security was enacted. Medicare and Medicaid, despite evidence of waste and inefficiency, have greatly enhanced the availability of quality health care to particularly vulnerable segments of the population. As we said at the outset, the challenge is to retain these remarkable accomplishments while bringing the growing costs of these programs under control.

Social Security

Social Security is the easiest of the programs to fix. After all, it operates by laws that transfer money from workers to retirees. If the costs must be reined in, the laws have to be changed. We have offered two primary mechanisms for bringing these costs under control.

First, change the way initial benefits are indexed. Currently, starting benefits rise with the average wage in the economy. The cost-saving alternative is to have these benefits go up with prices instead of wages. That switch alone would completely restore solvency to Social Security and then some. Note that such price indexing preserves the real value of the payroll tax amounts attributed to each beneficiary. We also think that progressive price indexing, a hybrid of wage and price indexing, is an attractive method for achieving Social Security reform. It offers wage indexing for those with low lifetime earnings, price indexing for those with high lifetime earnings, and a mix of the two for those in between.

Second, the system needs to recognize the steady but dramatic improvements in life expectancy and age-specific health that have been made over the past decades. It is not financially feasible in the twenty-first century for Americans to spend all their extra healthy years of life in retirement. The age at which people can collect full Social Security benefits and the earliest age at which they can receive benefits should be periodically or automatically adjusted upward.

We see many advantages to individual accounts. They would likely increase the national saving rate, they could replace the failed trust fund system, they would have all Americans participating in financial markets, and they would improve the adequacy of benefits. They can be part of the solution, but the real work on costs needs to be borne by two forms of indexing, one for prices and the other for increased life expectancy.

Providing adequate income for the elderly is a goal that can be accomplished. The provision of tax-advantaged status to individual or employer-sponsored contributions to retirement accounts will make the job easier. The Social Security system, the safety net for all Americans, can be transformed to ensure its solvency. The current rate of increase in benefit levels for people in the bottom third of the income distribution can be maintained, and the advantages of personal accounts can be merged readily into the system. The result: a system that is solvent, fair, and dependable. Delay is the enemy of ease and affordability of transition to this improved system. Congress must get to work.

A Healthy America

One of the principal reasons for increasing longevity is that the American people, on the whole, are healthier than ever. Better health is attributable, in large part, to the vast increase in knowledge about how the human body works, the impact of lifestyles on health, the massive research and development efforts on medications that treat diseases, and the vast improvements in medical practice. The system that produces these results, interactively on a world scale but with leadership from the United States, is a complex network of public and private efforts. Basic research is the key, and funding comes largely from private foundations and the federal government, especially the National Institutes of Health. Pharmaceutical and biotechnology companies have built upon basic research conducted in universities with dramatic results. This system needs to be preserved and enhanced.

There is a growing conviction in this country that everyone should have the opportunity for access to the health care system. That opportunity has been growing, just as the structure of the health care system has been undergoing important changes. But the costs are out of control.

Bringing health care costs under control is a tough challenge. But the first step is to recognize that they *are* out of control and understand what has caused the problem. A key part of the answer is simple economics. When people buy goods and services that are paid for either entirely or in large part by someone else, they generally are not wise shoppers in terms of seeking value for money. As Milton Friedman taught us, people never spend other people's money as carefully as their own. Moreover, health care is treated differently from any other part of the economy; in many ways, it has not been subject to budget constraints.

By this time, the vast majority of Americans are covered by some form of health insurance or are enrolled in one of the many health care organizations. Historically, the system has been structured in such a way that individuals become entitled to benefits without being sensitive to the costs of those benefits. One result has been massive inefficiency and poor allocation of resources. Another result has been a system dominated by providers and financiers of health care—in effect, a stool with only two legs. Reactions to these results have arisen at federal and state levels and among private employers and individuals. What these efforts reveal is the construction of a consumer leg on the unstable two-legged stool. As the consumer leg develops, the stool becomes sturdier, and the prospect for greater effectiveness in the use of resources increases. This is the key to controlling costs while maintaining access to health care for everyone.

Our proposals would give everyone the opportunity to have access to the health care system in an organized way. But price or available money would be factors in making health care decisions, as in the case of food, housing, transportation, clothing, or any of the other necessities of life. At some point in the future, preferably sooner rather than later, health care spending will have to be subject to the same value-for-money calculation that applies to everything else in the economy. The challenge is to limit spending, or at least the growth in spending, without curtailing medical advances and losing the benefits of modern medicine. Socially we need to sustain the high return of medical treatments and rein in waste and low-return activities.

An essential step toward containing health spending, particularly in Medicare and Medicaid, is to transform benefits from services to money. That is, the obligation that is now defined in terms of an open-ended entitlement to medical services would be converted to an obligation defined in terms of money. Money could take the form of medical vouchers that would ensure the ability of all participants in these programs to afford quality health care. They also would have choice regarding how that money is spent. For example, some might choose to buy comprehensive insurance while others might opt for major medical insurance plus Health Savings Accounts.

Another important step would control the growth in the aggregate value of Medicare and Medicaid vouchers, most naturally as a percentage of aggregate labor income. The essence of the cost problem is that the increase in health spending has been growing, and is projected to continue to grow, faster than labor earnings. This imbalance cannot continue forever. Vouchers would allow the government to gain more control over the growth in spending because an established amount of health care buying power would replace an open-ended entitlement to services. The era in which the government can promise Americans access to every medical treatment that might work cannot last. This is not radical thinking; everything else in the economy is rationed today by the market system, the best rationing system ever developed. People acquire what they want limited by what they can afford. That same logic will apply to health care. Americans will have the health care system they want and will choose the services most valuable to them, but they must be limited by what they can afford.

Developments consistent with this approach are traced in chapter 9, and important areas for further action are identified. Health Savings Accounts, created by federal legislation in 2003, are an essential building block. They can be useful to individuals, to state and local governments, and to employers. States are using the opportunity afforded by federal legislation to change their Medicaid programs, with broad movement toward bringing the consumer more directly into the process of choosing among alternative routes to health care. In chapter 10, we propose and show how to manage a shift toward vouchers in the structure of Medicare.

A strong third leg for the health care stool requires more than consumers who are empowered with the resources to buy their own health care; it also needs consumers who are well informed about prices and outcomes. This kind of information is now becoming available, largely in response to consumer demand, and those with the information have recognized that they must find a way to make it accessible. More work in this area is essential.

Competition among providers of the various forms of health insurance is also essential. Evidence is over-whelming that the present system, which prevents health insurance from being written on a national basis and bars consumers in one state from purchasing insurance in another, has led to startling differences in costs. Necessary legislative change has been clearly identified, and the battle among interests vested in the present system is in full swing. This battle must be won if the health insurance problem is to be resolved.

Continued movement in the directions now under way accompanied by actions on the recommendations put forward in chapter 10 can create a system of access to health care that is far superior to the existing system. The goal of universal opportunity for access to health care is achievable with costs that, though certainly substantial, will not be of the runaway nature that is commonly projected for the current system.

The recommendations presented here constitute a plan of action to modernize our entitlement programs in keeping with today's opportunities and results. The challenge, though difficult, can—and must—be met. Let us get on with the job.

APPENDIX

Entitlement Reform at a Glance

ENTITLEMENT REFORM AT A GLANCE

1. Make a Big Pie
2. Income for Retirement
3. A Healthy America
4. Containing the Costs

1. Make a Big Pie

Keep the economy strong:

- Retain flexibility.
- Control inflation.
- Keep tax rates low.
- Encourage private saving.
- Balance the federal budget at full employment.
- Strive to reduce income inequality.
- Encourage participation in the labor force by changing incentives to work.
  - Encourage work with low tax rates.
  - Count top forty years of earnings for Social Security.
  - Consider a worker to be paid up after forty years for Social Security.
  - Remove the high 46 percent tax rate on some Social Security recipients.
  - Improve incentives for long careers by changing the formula for high-income but short-career beneficiaries.
  - Make Medicare the primary payer, thereby making older workers more attractive as employees.
  - Change Medicaid system to remove the present disincentive to work.

2. Income for Retirement

Promote policies that encourage private pension plans:

- Portable plans
- Employers matching employees' contributions
- Automatic enrollment
- Automatic investment of tax refunds in IRAs

Solvent Alternatives for Social Security

- Progressive Price Indexing Plus plan
  - Keep wage indexing for lowest 30 percent.
  - Phase in price indexing for those at higher levels of lifetime earnings.
  - Index age of full benefits to longevity changes.
- Personal Security Account plan
  - Combine $600 flat benefit that is wage indexed with 5 percent individual accounts (2.5 percent new contribution matched by Social Security).
  - Index age of full benefits to longevity changes.
- President's Commission on Social Security: Reform Model 2
  - Switch to price indexing with funds devoted to new minimum for low-income workers.
  - Provide an option to redirect up to 4 percent of payroll tax to personal accounts up to $1,000 per year.
  - Enhance contribution by low-income beneficiaries to private accounts.
  - Consider additional options:
    —Remove dollar cap on private accounts.
    —Combine with matched 2.5 percentage points of payroll tax.
    —Index age of full benefits to longevity changes.
- Emanuel plan
  - Introduce Universal Savings Accounts.
  - Invest a matched 1 percent of payroll tax in "life cycle funds."
- Feldstein and Samwick plan
  - Reduce current benefit levels gradually by 40 percent.
  - Invest a matched 1.5 percentage points in private accounts.
- Peter G. Peterson plan
  - Switch to price indexing with add-on personal accounts and safety net for low-income workers.
- Diamond and Orszag plan
  - Achieve long-run solvency through a combination of benefit reductions and tax increases.

3. A Healthy America

Americans are living longer, healthier lives. To continue in this direction:

- Support basic research and development.
- Make available information on the effects of lifestyle on health.
- Create a system in which informed consumers are given choices of health care.
- Encourage a system in which consumers have more fiscal responsibility for their health care.

Private system

- Encourage national, rather than state, insurance competition.
- Inform consumers about health service prices and quality.
- Strengthen incentives for company-sponsored HSAs and catastrophic insurance.
- Make tax-advantaged HSAs and low-cost catastrophic insurance available to all who do not have employer-sponsored plans.

Medicare

- Risk-adjusted vouchers
- Consumer choice
- Smart means testing
- Gradual transition to new program
- Financing within the constraint of a balanced budget at full employment

Medicaid

- Risk-adjusted vouchers
- States allowed to experiment with structure
- Consumer choice
- Increased coverage, replacing eligibility notch with gradual reduction of the value of vouchers
- Disciplined federal support by a commitment to a balanced budget at full employment

4. Containing the Costs

Social Security

- Price indexing or progressive price indexing will keep benefit levels within revenues from existing payroll tax.
- Indexing age of full benefits to longevity further improves solvency.
- Adequacy can be strengthened by use of personal accounts on a carve-out or add-on basis or a combination of the two.
- Retain or enhance progressivity.

Health

- Arrange Medicare and Medicaid systems so that entitlements are defined in terms of monetary contributions rather than services.
- Replace obligations that are open-ended with obligations that have an identified cost.
- Support a commitment to a balanced budget at full employment.
- Encourage competition between insurers or health care providers.
- Permit insurance to be written on a national basis.
- Make HSAs available to individuals on their own and make associated insurance portable across state lines.
- Inform and empower consumers, who will have a profound impact on reform.

These steps provide useful building blocks for private employers and state and city governments, and the associated consumer involvement will lower costs.

Notes

Introduction

1. Steven R. Weisman, "Fed Chief Warns That Entitlement Growth Could Harm Economy," *New York Times*, January 19, 2007, C1.
2. Peter G. Peterson, *Running on Empty* (New York: Farrar, Straus and Giroux, 2004), and Laurence J. Kotlikoff, "Is the United States Bankrupt?," *Federal Reserve Bank of St. Louis Review* (July–August 2006).
3. Congressional Budget Office, "The Long Term Budget Outlook," December 2005, available at http://www.cbo.gov/ftpdocs/69xx/doc6982/12-15-LongTermOutlook.pdf, accessed December 19, 2007. Office of Management and Budget, "Budget of the United States Government Fiscal Year 2005: Historical Tables," Table 1.2, available at http://www.whitehouse.gov/omb/budget/fy2005/ hist .html, accessed December 19, 2007.

Chapter 1. A Story of Success: Healthy People in a Healthy Economy

1. Marc Bloom, "At 73, Marathoner Runs as If He's Stopped the Clock," *New York Times*, February 12, 2005, D6.
2. Author's calculation based on life tables from 2004 Social Security Trustees Report.
3. Federal Interagency Forum on Aging-Related Statistics, *Older Americans 2004: Key Indicators of Well-Being*, Table 19A.
4. Ibid., Table 26A.
5. Ibid., Table 25.
6. Ibid., Table 20.

7. In his Nobel lecture, "The Transformation of Macroeconomic Policy and Research," Prescott said:

Good statistics are available on labor supply and tax rates across the major advanced industrial countries. My measure of aggregate labor supply is aggregate hours worked in the market sector divided by the number of working-age people. Given that the effect of the marginal effective tax rate on labor supply depends on this elasticity, and given that tax rates vary considerably, these observations provide an almost ideal test of whether the aggregate labor supply elasticity is 3. The set of countries that Prescott (2004) studied are the G-7 countries, which are the large advanced industrial countries. The differences in marginal tax rates and labor supply are large: Canada, Japan, and the United States have rates near 0.40, and France, Germany, and Italy near 0.60. The prediction, based on an aggregate labor supply elasticity of 3, that Western Europeans will work one-third less than North Americans and Japanese, is confirmed. Added evidence for an aggregate elasticity of 3 is that it explains why labor supply in France and Germany was nearly 50 percent greater during the 1970–74 period than it is today. Observations on aggregate labor supply across countries and across time imply a labor supply elasticity near 3.

Journal of Political Economy 114, no. 2 (April 2006), 225.

8. Joseph A. Schumpeter, *Capitalism, Socialism, and Democracy* (New York: Harper & Row, 1942).

9. Bureau of Labor Statistics, Series BDS00000000000000 00110001LQ5 and BDS0000000000000000110004LQ5.

10. Ibid.

11. U.S. Census Bureau, *The 2006 Statistical Abstract*, Table 743.

12. Dow Jones, "Dow Jones Industrial Average History," accessible at http://djindexes.com/mdsidx/downloads/DJIA_Hist_Comp .pdf.

13. Bureau of Economic Analysis, *U.S. International Transaction Accounts Data*.

Chapter 2. The Iceberg Ahead

1. Rudolph G. Penner and C. Eugene Steuerle, "Budget Crisis at the Door," *Urban Institute Brief*, October 2003.

2. "The Long-Term Budget Outlook, December 2005," Congress of the United States, Congressional Budget Office, 43.

3. *The 2007 Annual Report of the Board of Trustees of the Federal Old-Age and Survivors Insurance and Federal Disability Insurance Trust Funds*, 2.

4. Ibid.

5. John Goodman, testimony before House Committee on Ways and Means, May 19, 2005.

6. Ben Bernanke, quoted in "Fed Chief Warns That Entitlement Growth Could Harm Economy," *New York Times*, January 19, 2007, C1.

7. "The Budget and Economic Outlook: Fiscal Years 2006 to 2015," Congressional Budget Office, January 25, 2005, Appendix F, Table 2.

8. Office of Budget and Management, "Budget of the United States Government Fiscal Year 2007: Historical Tables," Table 1.2, available at http://www.whitehouse.gov/omb/budget/fy2007/hist.html, access December 19, 2007.

9. Aon Consulting, "State of Maryland: Postemployment Benefits Other than Pension Actuarial Valuation," October 2005.

10. Mary Williams Walsh, "$58 Billion Shortfall for New Jersey Retiree Care," *New York Times*, July 25, 2007, A1.

11. California Legislative Analyst's Office, "Analysis of the 2005–06 Budget Bill: School District Financial Condition," February 2005.

12. "Pension Woes," *San Diego Union-Tribune*, January 7, 2006, A17.

13. Elliott Spagat, "San Diego Mayor Resigns in Midst of Federal Probe of City Hall," Associated Press, April 25, 2005.

14. "City Gets a Sobering Look at Possible Pension Trouble," *New York Times*, August 20, 2006, A1.

15. Calculation based on National Association of State Budget Officers, *2003 State Expenditure Report*.

16. Defined benefit programs promise retirement benefits based on years of service and salary levels rather than on contributions and investment returns.

17. Chris Foreman, "Saving General Motors," *System Contractor News*, May 1, 2006.

18. Centers for Medicare and Medicaid Services, "National Health Expenditures Aggregate and Per Capita Amounts, Percent Distribution, and Average Annual Percent Growth, by Source of Funds: Selected Calendar Years 1960–2004," http://www .cms.hhs.gov/NationalHealthExpendData/downloads/tables.pdf. Centers for Medicare and Medicaid Services, "National Health Care Expenditure Projections: 2004–2014," http://www.cms.hhs .gov/NationalHealthExpendData/downloads/nheprojections 2004–2014.pdf.

19. Centers for Medicare and Medicaid Services, "National Health Care Expenditure Data," http://www.cms.hhs.gov/National HealthExpendData/.

20. T. M. Selden and B. M. Gray, "Tax Subsidies for Employment-Related Health Insurance: Estimates for 2006," *Health Affairs* 25, no. 6, (November 1, 2006), 1568–79.

Chapter 3. Age and the Labor Force

1. Author's calculation based on life tables from 2004 Social Security Trustees Report.

2. Each year of earnings is subject to a wage indexing factor under current law. The Social Security benefit calculation is described in more detail in chapter 5.

3. In addition to the income taxation of Social Security benefits, there is the complicated issue of the so-called earnings test. If Social Security beneficiaries are younger than the age of full-retirement benefits (currently sixty-six), then each dollar of labor earnings exceeding $13,560 causes their Social Security benefits to be lowered by $0.50. While there is some recalculation of subsequent benefits after reaching the full retirement age, this earnings test clearly discourages work effort. Fortunately, it does not apply to those older than the full retirement age.

Chapter 4. Income for Retirement

1. U.S. Department of Labor, Pension and Welfare Benefits Administration, *Private Pension Plan Bulletin* (Spring 1999, Winter 2001–2002, July 2005, July 2006). Tables E1, E8 and A1.

2. CBO, *The Risk Exposure of the Pension Benefit Guaranty Corporation*, September 2004.

3. Brigitte C. Madrian and Dennis F. Shea, "The Power of Suggestion: Inertia in 401(k) Participation and Savings Behavior," *Quarterly Journal of Economics* 116, no. 4 (November 2001), 1149–87.

4. Arthur H. Vandenberg, "The $47,000,000,000 Blight," *Saturday Evening Post* 209, no. 43 (April 24, 1937), 5–7.

5. Bill Clinton, remarks on Social Security at Georgetown University, Washington, DC, February 9, 1998.

Chapter 5. Principles for Reforming Social Security

1. In addition to the 6.20 percent Social Security payroll tax, both the employer and the employee face a 1.45 percent payroll tax for Medicare. Unlike the Social Security tax, the Medicare tax applies to all earnings rather than just to a capped amount ($97,500 in 2007).

2. In order to qualify for any retirement benefit at all, one has to have at least forty quarters (or ten years) of covered employment.

3. This can be explained even more explicitly with some simple arithmetic. Let W be the average wage, B the average Social Security benefit, T the tax rate, Nr the number of retirees, and Nw the number of workers. Therefore, if we have a pure pay-as-you-go program, at any point in time expense must equal revenue and $Nr \times B = W \times T \times Nw$. Rearranging the equation, we have $(B/W) \times T = (Nr/Nw)$. (B/W) is roughly constant because of wage indexing, and if life expectancy gains cause the dependency ratio (Nr/Nw) to increase, then the tax rate must also increase. If life expectancy is constantly expanding and the length of retirement grows longer, then wage indexing causes a never-ending series of tax shortfalls.

4. House of Commons, Social Security Committee, *Social Security—Seventh Report*: 2000. Session 1999–2000, section 55.

5. Daniele Franco, "Italy: A Never-Ending Pension Reform," and

Didier Blanchet and Florence Legros, "France: The Difficult Path to Consensual Reforms," in *Social Security Pension Reform in Europe*, ed. Martin Feldstein and Horst Siebert (Chicago: University of Chicago Press, 2002).

6. Axel Borsh-Supan and Christina B. Wilke, "The German Public Pension System: How It Was, How It Will Be." NBER Working Paper 10525, May 2004.

7. Summary of the 2006 Trustees Report, Social Security and Medicare Board of Trustees.

Chapter 6. Plans for Reforming Social Security

1. Its principal component is the same as the Pozen plan described in Richard Pozen, Sylvester J. Schieber, and John B. Shoven, "Improving Social Security's Progressivity and Solvency with Hybrid Indexing," *American Economic Review* 94, no. 2 (May 1, 2004), 187–91.

2. It is an updated version of the PSA 2000 plan described in Sylvester J. Schieber and John B. Shoven, "Administering a Cost Effective National Program of Personal Security Accounts," in *Administrative Aspects of Investment-Based Social Security Reform*, ed. John B. Shoven (Chicago: University of Chicago Press, 2000).

3. "Strengthening Social Security and Creating Personal Wealth for All Americans," Final Report of the President's Commission to Strengthen Social Security, December 21, 2001.

4. Ibid., 119.

5. Rahm Emanuel, "Supplementing Social Security," *Wall Street Journal*, September 13, 2007, A17.

6. Martin Feldstein and Andrew Samwick, "Potential Paths of Social Security Reform," *Tax Policy and Economy 2001*, ed. James Poterba (Cambridge, MA.: MIT Press), 181–224.

Chapter 7. The Past Is Prologue

1. OECD Health Data 2006.

2. Kaiser Family Foundation, *2006 Kaiser/HRET Employer Health Benefits Survey*, 2.

3. E. S. Fisher, D. E. Wennberg, T. A. Stukel, D. J. Gottlieb, F. L. Lucas, and E. L. Pinder, "The Implications of Regional Variations in Medicare Spending. Part 1: The Content, Quality, and Accessibility of Care," *Annals of Internal Medicine* (2003), 273–87.

4. ABC News/Kaiser Family Foundation/USA Today, *Health Care in America Survey*, September 2003.

5. We have benefited greatly from Milton Friedman, "How to Cure Health Care," *Public Interest* (Winter 2001); John F. Cogan, R. Glenn Hubbard, and Daniel P. Kessler, *Healthy, Wealthy, & Wise: Five Steps to a Better Health Care System* (Washington, DC: AEI Press, and Stanford, CA: Hoover Institution, 2005); Michael F. Cannon and Michael D. Tanner, *Healthy Competition* (Washington, DC: Cato Institute, 2005); Michael E. Porter and Elizabeth Olmsted Teisberg, *Redefining Health Care: Creating Value-Based Competition on Results* (Cambridge, MA: Harvard Business School Press, 2006); and John Goodman and Gerald Musgrove, *Patient Power* (Washington, DC: Cato Institute, 1993).

6. Melissa A. Thomasson, "From Sickness to Health: The Twentieth Century Development of U.S. Health Insurance," *Explorations in Economic History* 39, no. 3 (July 2002), 233–53.

7. Employers did not initially report the value of these fringe benefits to the Internal Revenue Service as wages. This tax exemption became part of the revenue code in 1954, thereby clearing up any ambiguity about this large subsidy.

8. Kaiser Family Foundation, *Employer Health Benefits: 2005 Annual Survey*, 1.

9. Table 1, http://www.kff.org/medicaid/upload/kcmu032106full.pdf.

10. Amy J. Davidoff, Garrett Bowen, and Matthew Schirmer, "Children Eligible for Medicaid but Not Enrolled," Urban Institute, September 2000.

11. Amy J. Davidoff, Bowen Garrett, and Alshadye Yemane, "Medicaid-Eligible Adults Who Are Not Enrolled: Who Are They and Do They Get the Care They Need?" (Washington, DC: Urban Institute, October 2001, http://www.urban.org/url .cfm?ID+310378, accessed January 9, 2008.

12. The United States, including the District of Columbia and Puerto Rico, and the U.S. territories of American Samoa, Guam, the Northern Mariana Islands, and the Virgin Islands all have separate Medicaid programs.

13. Kaiser Family Foundation, "Medicaid's Role for Women," November 2004.

14. Kaiser Family Foundation, "Medicaid Enrollment and Spending Trends," May 2006.

15. Kaiser Family Foundation, "Medicaid and Long-Term Care Services," July 2006.

16. Ibid.

17. 2007 Annual Report of the Boards of Trustees of the Federal Hospital Insurance and Federal Supplementary Medical Insurance Trust Funds, 34.

18. This characterization is drawn from Porter and Teisberg, op. cit.

19. Clifford J. Levy and Michael Luo, "New York Medicaid Fraud May Reach into Billions," *New York Times*, July 18, 2005, A1.

20. Ibid.

21. John E. Wennberg, Elliott S. Fisher, and Jonathan S. Skinner, "Geography and the Debate over Medicare Reform," *Health Affairs*, Web Exclusive.

22. Ibid., 15.

23. Joseph Newhouse and the Insurance Experiment Group, *Free for All? Lessons from the RAND Health Insurance Experiment* (Cambridge, MA: Harvard University Press, 1993), 243.

24. Arnold Milstein, M.D., in testimony before the Senate Health, Education, Labor and Pensions Committee, January 28, 2004.

Chapter 8. How to Improve Health Care

1. Sir Alexander Fleming, "Penicillin," Nobel lecture, December 11, 1945, http://nobelprize.org/nobel_prizes/medicine/laureates /1945/fleming-lecture.html.

2. Ernst B. Chain, "The Chemical Structure of the Penicillins," Nobel lecture, March 20, 1946, http://nobelprize.org/nobel _prizes/medicine/laureates/1945/chain-lecture.html.

3. Jonathan Myers, Ph.D., "Fitness, Physical Activity Patterns and

Health Outcomes." Presentation, Stanford University School of Medicine, Stanford, CA, December 7, 2005.

4. Todd M. Manini, James E. Everhart, Kushang V. Patel, Dale A. Schoeller, Lisa H. Colbert, Marjolein Visser, Frances Tylavsky, Douglas C. Bauer, Bret H. Goodpaster, and Tamara B. Harris, "Daily Activity Energy Expenditure and Mortality Among Older Adults," *JAMA* 296 (2006), 171–79.

5. Hamilton Moses III, E. Ray Dorsey, David H. M. Matheson, and Samuel O. Thier, "Financial Anatomy of Biomedical Research," *JAMA* 294 (2005), 1333–42.

6. David Gratzer, *The Cure: How Capitalism Can Save American Health Care* (New York: Encounter Books, 2006), 4.

7. William D. Nordhaus, "The Health of Nations: The Contribution of Improved Health to Living Standards," NBER Working Paper No. W8818 (March 2002).

8. Kevin M. Murphy and Robert H. Topel, *Measuring the Gains from Medical Research: An Economic Approach* (Chicago: University of Chicago Press, 2003), 3–4. For additional analysis of the relationship of increases in longevity and the emergence of new drugs, see Frank R. Lichtenberg, "Pharmaceutical Innovation, Mortality Reduction, and Economic Growth," Conference on the Economic Value of Medical Research, Washington, DC, December 2–3, 1999.

9. Kevin M. Murphy and Robert H. Topel, "The Value of Health and Longevity," *Journal of Political Economy* 115, no. 5 (2006), 871.

Chapter 9. First Steps Toward Change

1. Michael Cannon and Michael Tanner, *Healthy Competition: What's Holding Back Health Care and How to Free It* (Washington, DC: Cato Institute, 2005), 7–8.

2. Ibid.

3. Pew Internet and American Life Project, *Health Information Online* (May 2005).

4. Pew Internet and American Life Project, *Online Health Search 2005* (October 2006).

5. "Doctors Using Google to Diagnose Illnesses," *Daily Mail,*

November 10, 2006, http://www.dailymail.co.uk/pages/live
/articles/news/news.html?in_article_id=415562&in_page_id=1
770.

6. Christopher Bowe, "Walk-In Clinics Help to Cure US Health-
care Ills," *Financial Times*, December 6, 2007, http://www.ft
.com/cms/s/0/635b0292-a39e-11dc-b229-0000779fd2ac.html.

7. Jerome H. Grossman, M.D., "Physician's Work: How the
Evolution of Medicine and Supporting Technology Allows for Its
Transfer to Professional Staff and Benefits Patients" (Cambridge,
MA: Mossavar-Rahmani Center for Business and Government,
September 28, 2007), http://www.ksg.harvard.edu/m-rcbg/ hcdp/
readings/Periodic_Observations.pdf., accessed January 9, 2008.

8. "Aetna Expands Efforts to Provide Consumers with a
Transparent View of Health Care Costs and Quality,"
http://www.aetna.com/news/2006/pr_20060613.htm.

9. The Centers for Medicare and Medicaid Services (CMS)
recently released records on tens of thousands of heart defib-
rillator implants. The data showed that about 4 percent of
these patients had at least one complication during the
implant procedure. This percentage is within understood
boundaries identified in other studies. Other studies also have
shown a wide divergence of complications among doctors and
hospitals largely on the basis of the number of implants a doctor performs. The agency was concerned about making public
information about doctors since that might result in disclosing
patients' identities. Barry Meier, "U.S. Shields Doctor Data in
Implants," *New York Times*, July 10, 2006, C1.

10. Haneefa Saleem, "Health Spending Accounts," http://www
.bls.gov/opub/cwc/cm20031022ar01p1.htm, accessed June 29,
2007.

11. "Medical Savings Accounts: Obstacles to Their Growth and
Ways to Improve Them," National Center for Policy Analysis,
Policy Report 216, July 1998, http://www.ncpa.org/studies
/s216.html.

12. In order to make contributions to a Health Savings Account,
an employee must be enrolled in a qualifying high-deductible
health plan. If an employee is insured through a group plan

with his or her employer, then the health plan will not follow the worker if he or she switches jobs. If an individual moves to a different state, he or she may also need to switch health insurance.

13. Congressional Budget Office, Cost Estimate, S. 1932, Deficit Reduction Act of 2005, January 27, 2006, 34, http://www.cbo.gov/ftpdoc.cfm?index=7028&type=1.

14. Governor Mark Sanford, "Medicaid Reform Key to Better Outcomes, Slowing Growth," October 1, 2005, http://www.scgoveror.com/uploads/upload/NR-c111605-MedLetter.pdf.

15. Lucette Lagnado, "Seniors in Vermont Are Finding They Can Go Home Again," *Wall Street Journal*, October 23, 2006, A1.

16. "Medicare Advantage Plans Provide Lower Costs and Substantial Savings," Center for Medicare & Medicaid Services, April 3, 2006.

17. Sarah Lueck and Jane Zhang, "Give Us Your Sick," *Wall Street Journal*, October 21, 2006, R5.

18. Richard S. Foster, "Financial Status of Medicare," presentation for the American Enterprise Institute, April 24, 2007.

19. Daniel L. McFadden, "A Dog's Breakfast," *Wall Street Journal*, February 16, 2007, A15.

20. Kaiser Family Foundation, 2006 Kaiser/HRET *Employer Health Benefits Survey*.

Chapter 10. Medicare, Medicaid, and Health Care Reform

1. Milton Friedman, "How to Cure Health Care," *Public Interest* (Winter 2001), 21.

2. Ibid., 22.

3. Ezekiel J. Emanuel, M.D., Ph.D., and Victor R. Fuchs, Ph.D., "Health Care Vouchers: A Proposal for Universal Coverage," *New England Journal of Medicine* 352 (March 24, 2005), 1255–60.

4. John F. Cogan, R. Glenn Hubbard, and Daniel P. Kessler, *Healthy, Wealthy, and Wise* (Washington DC: AEI Press; and Stanford, CA: Hoover Institution Press, 2005).

5. Ibid., 82.

6. These numbers are as of January 2006, according to the GAO report "Consumer-Directed Health Plans: Small but Growing Enrollment Fueled by Rising Cost of Health Care Coverage," April 28, 2006.

7. Devon M. Herrick, "How to Create a Competitive Insurance Market," *National Center for Policy Analysis*, Brief Analysis No. 558 (June 15, 2006).

Chapter 11. Conclusions

1. Joseph A. Schumpeter, an Austrian, was a major economic thinker of the twentieth century who coined the phase "creative destruction."

2. Pension Protection Act of 2006, signed August 17, 2006.

Index